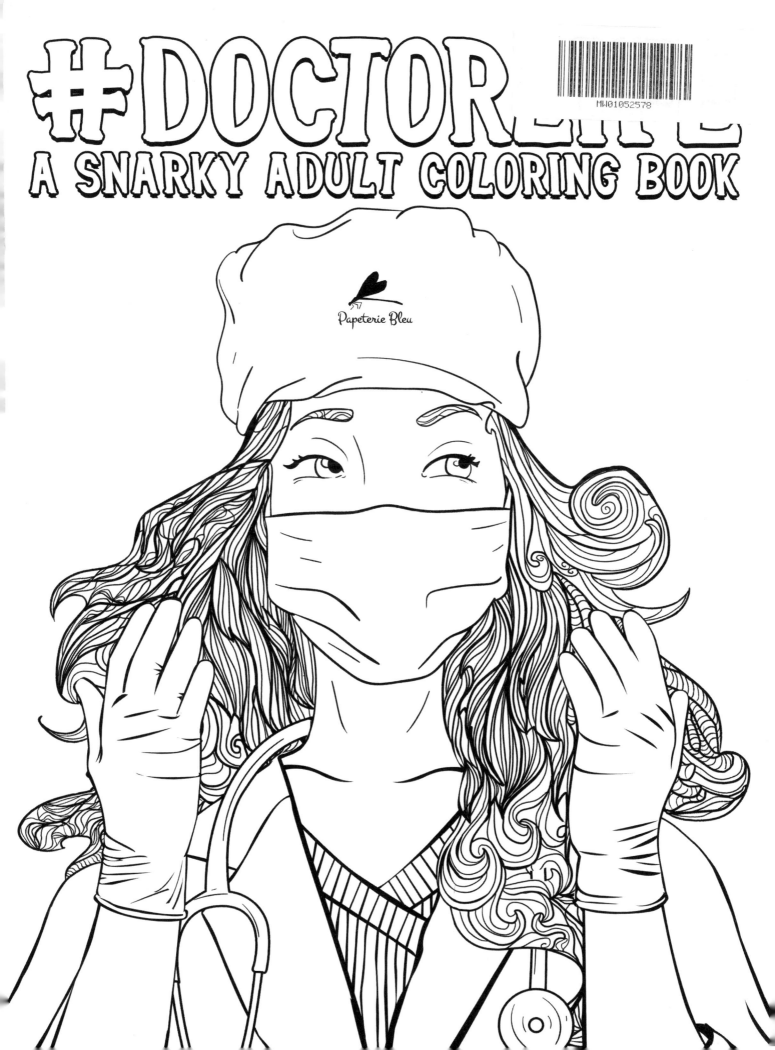

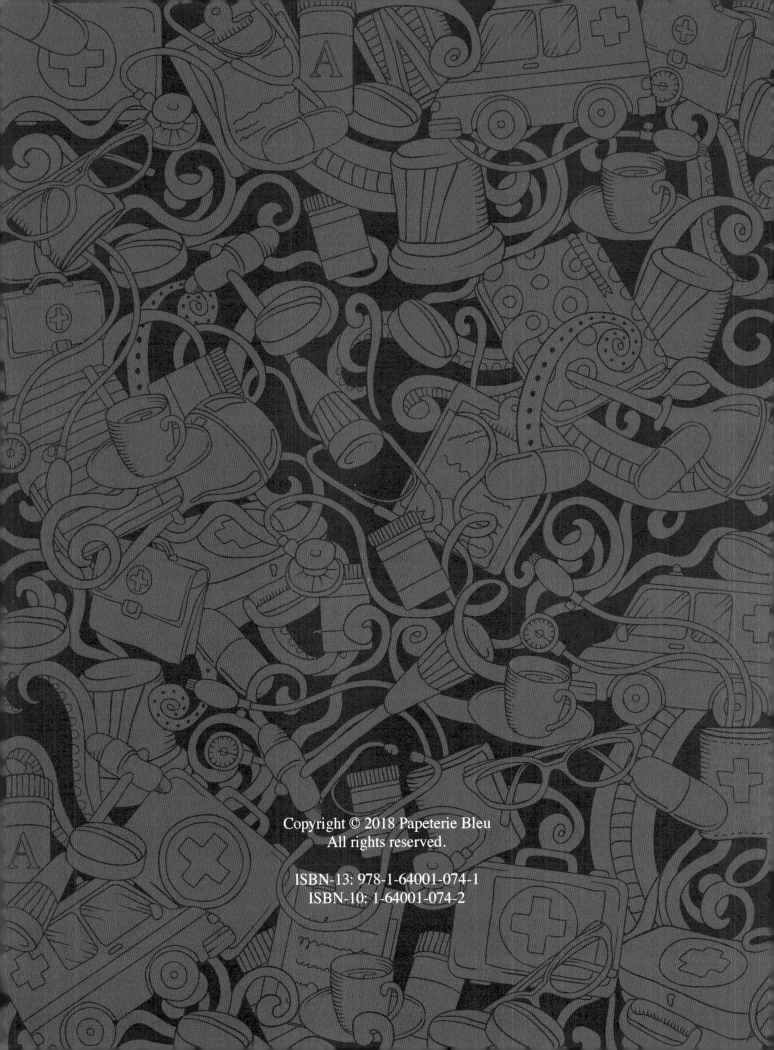

ISBN-13: 978-1-64001-074-1
ISBN-10: 1-64001-074-2

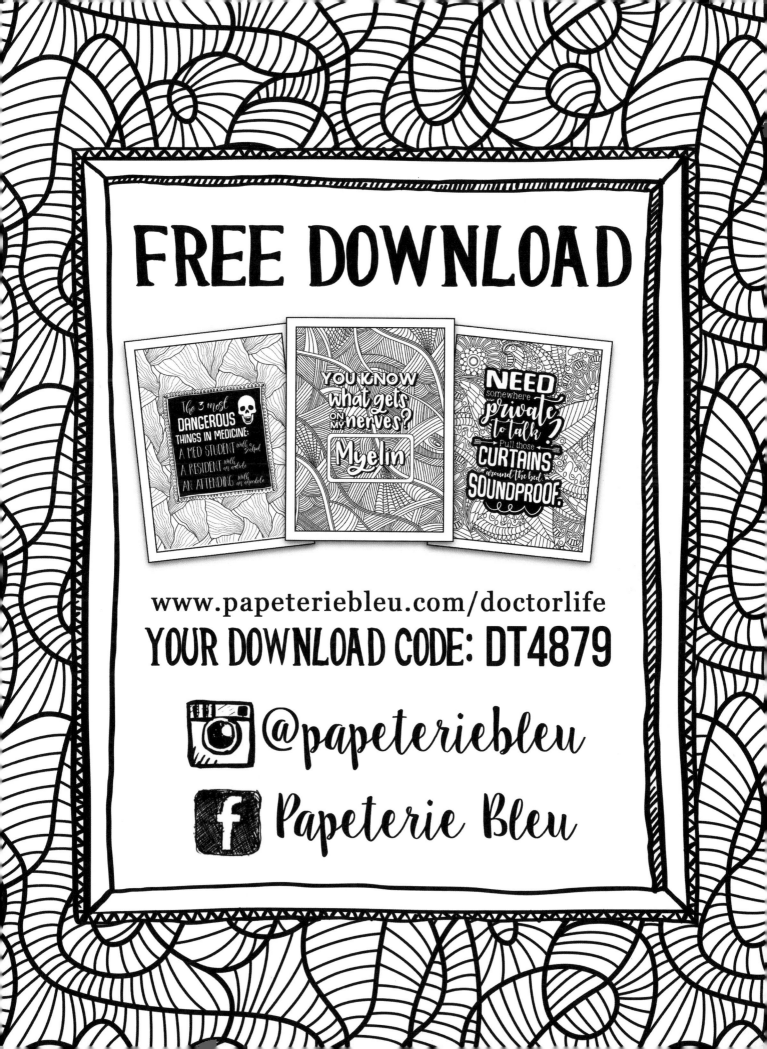

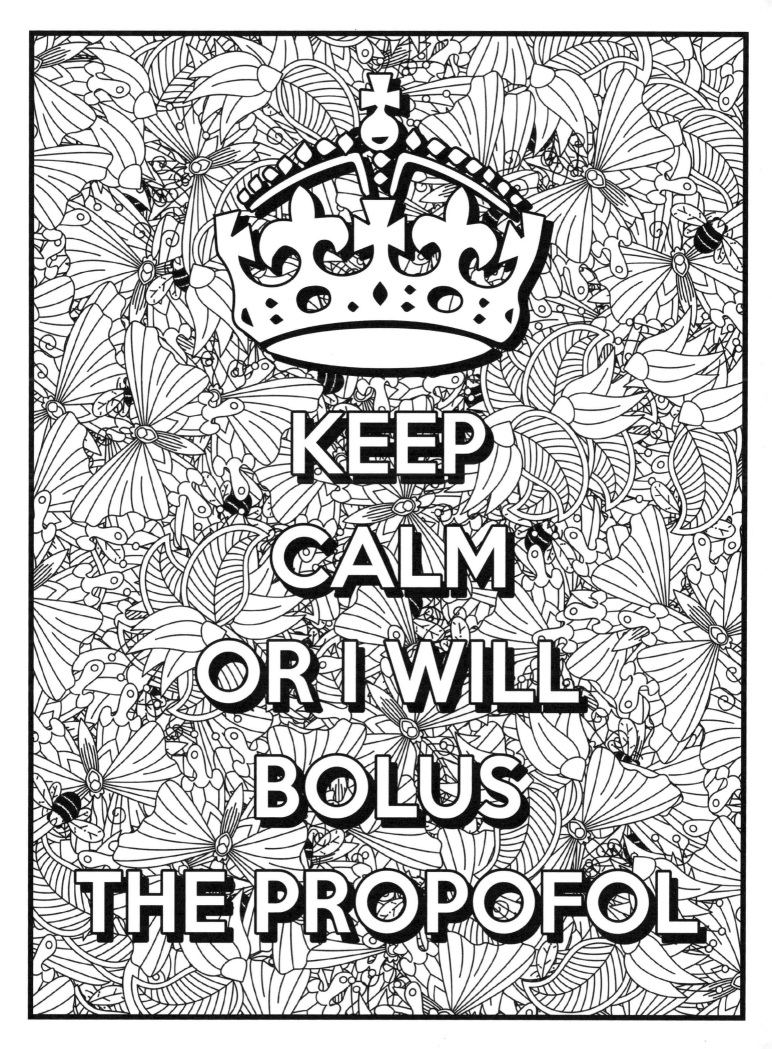

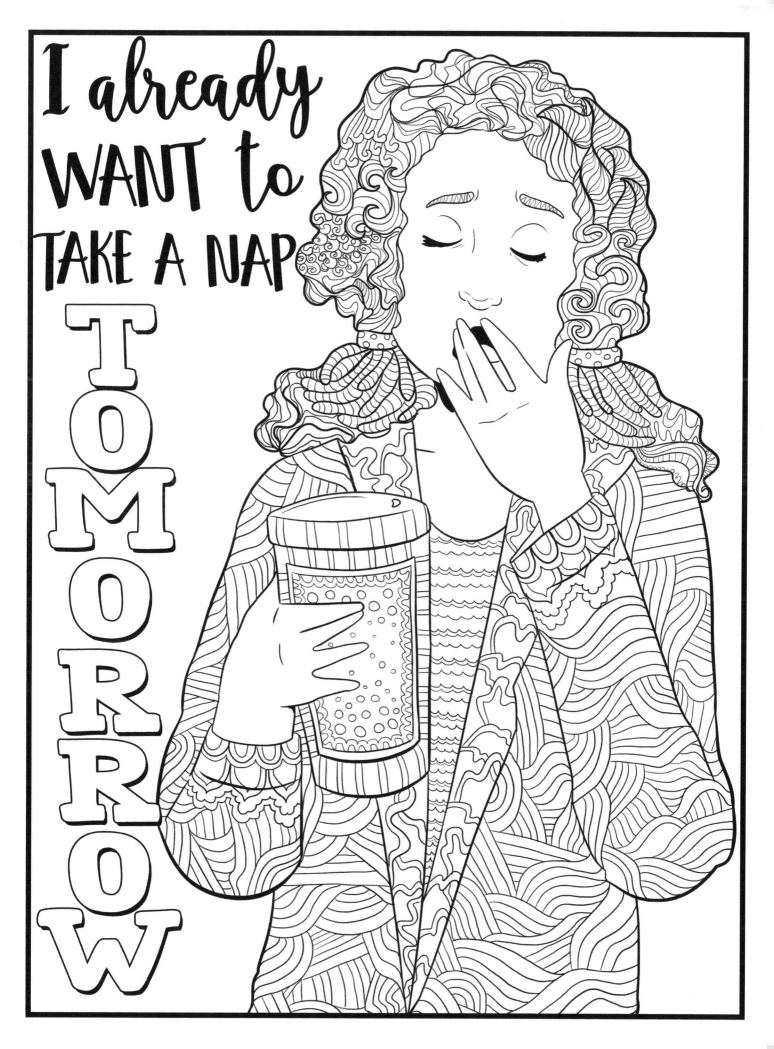

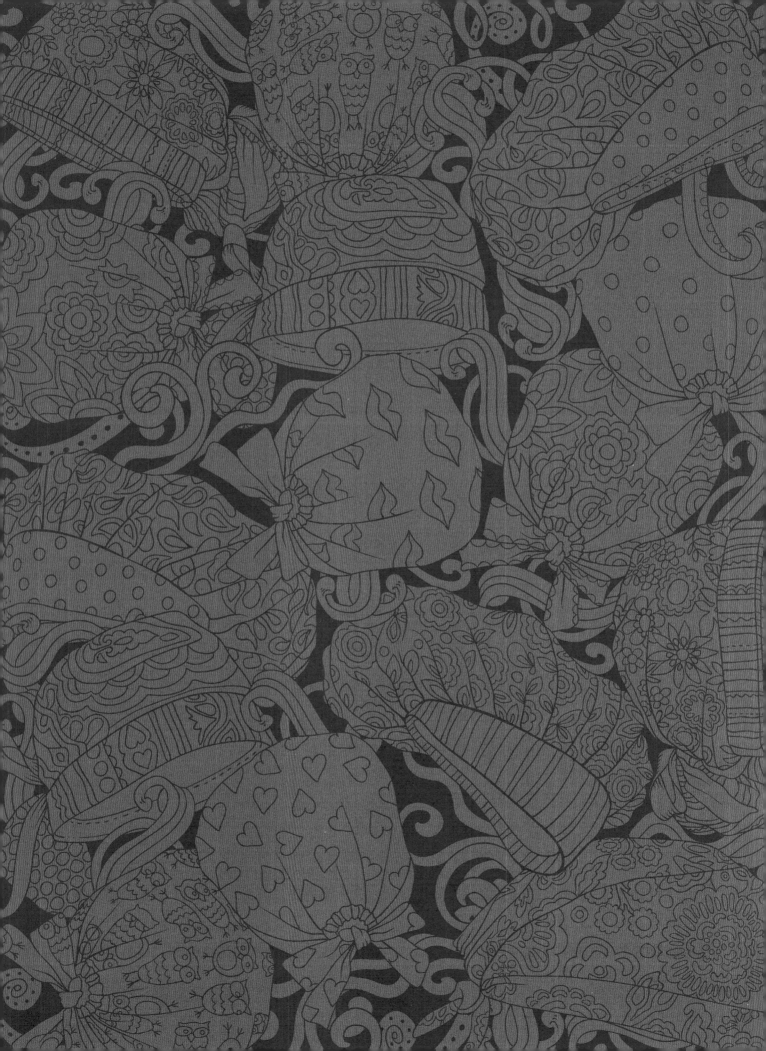

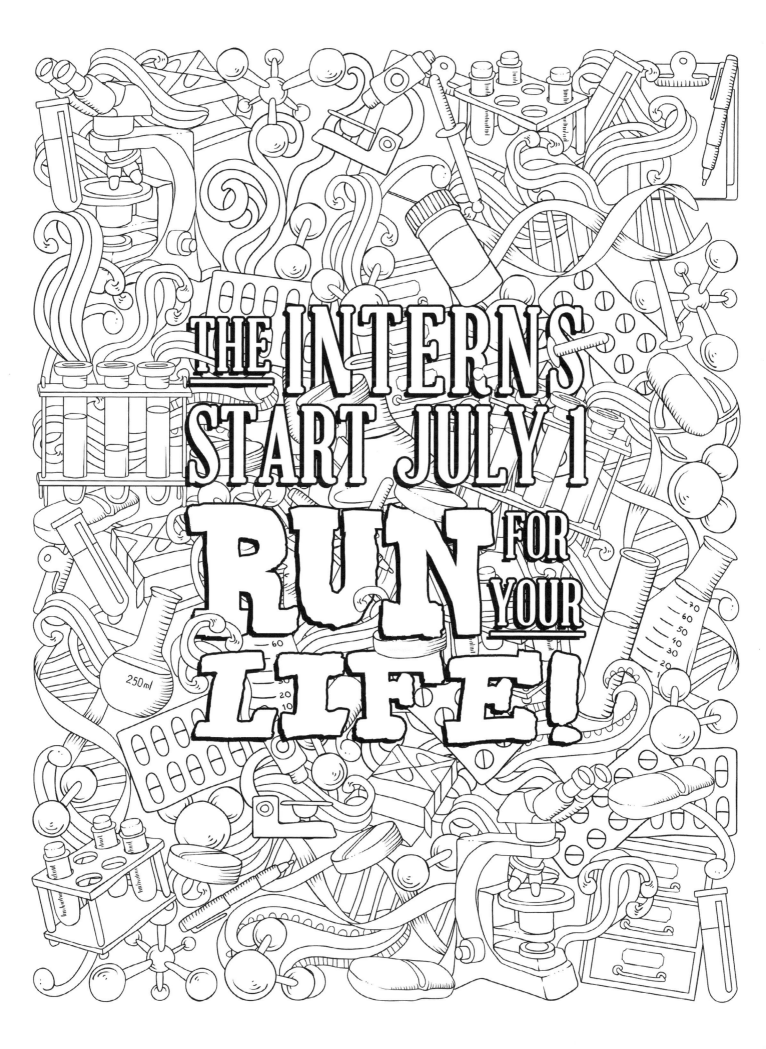

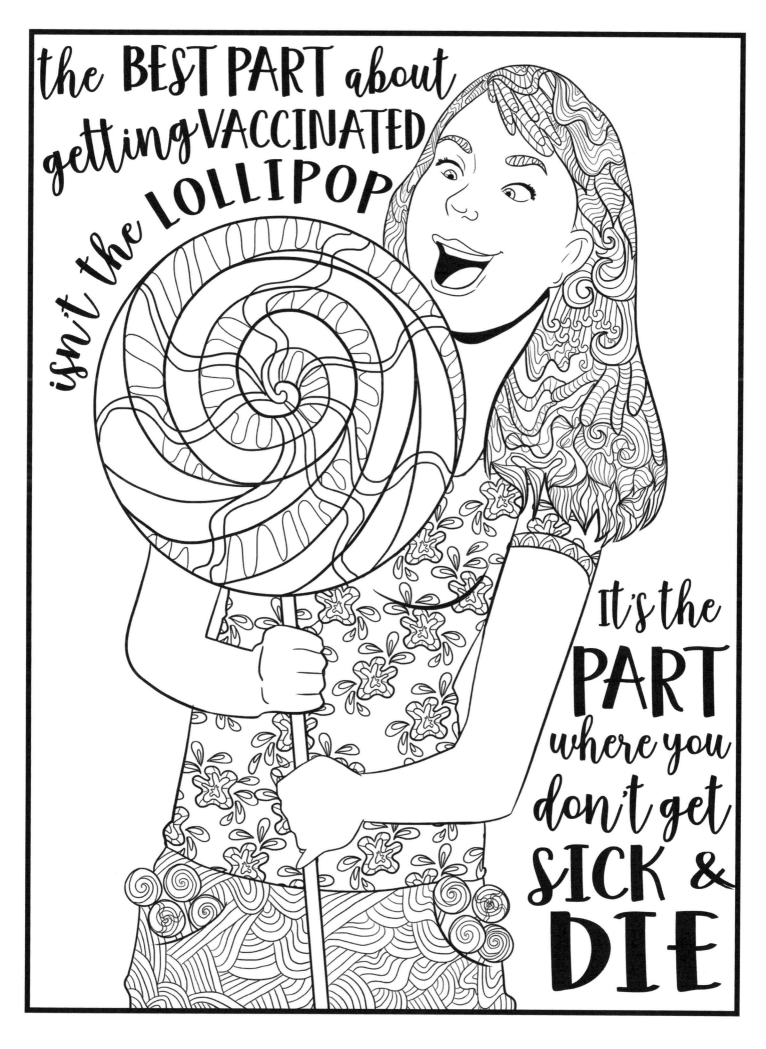

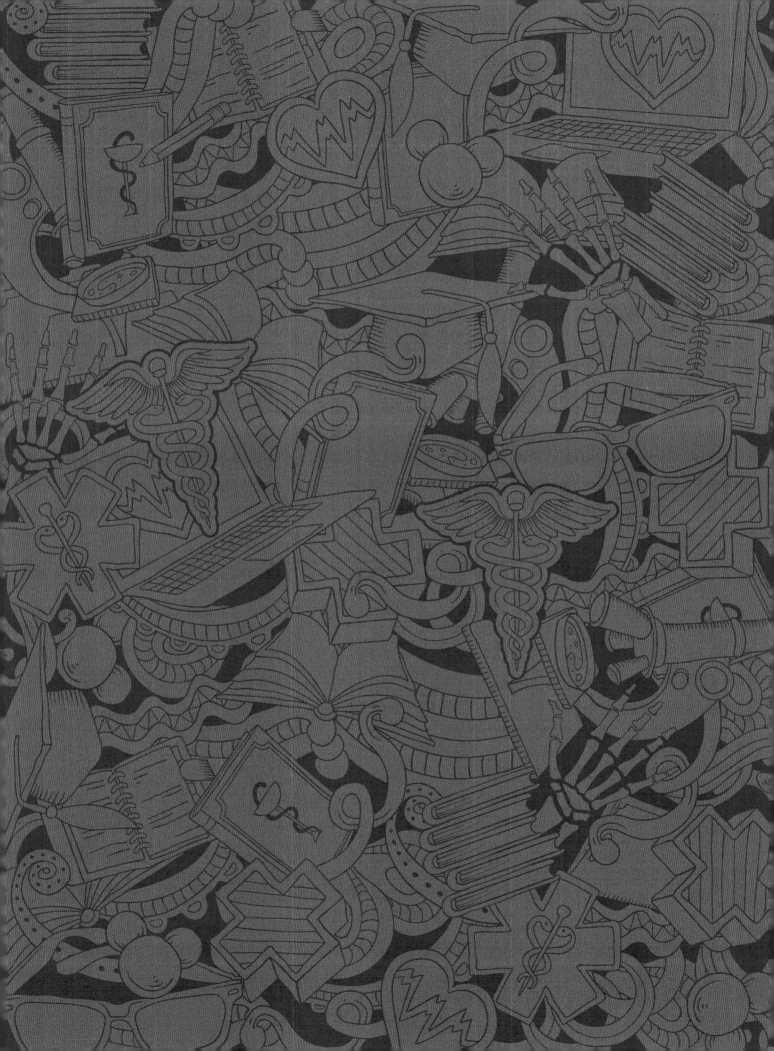

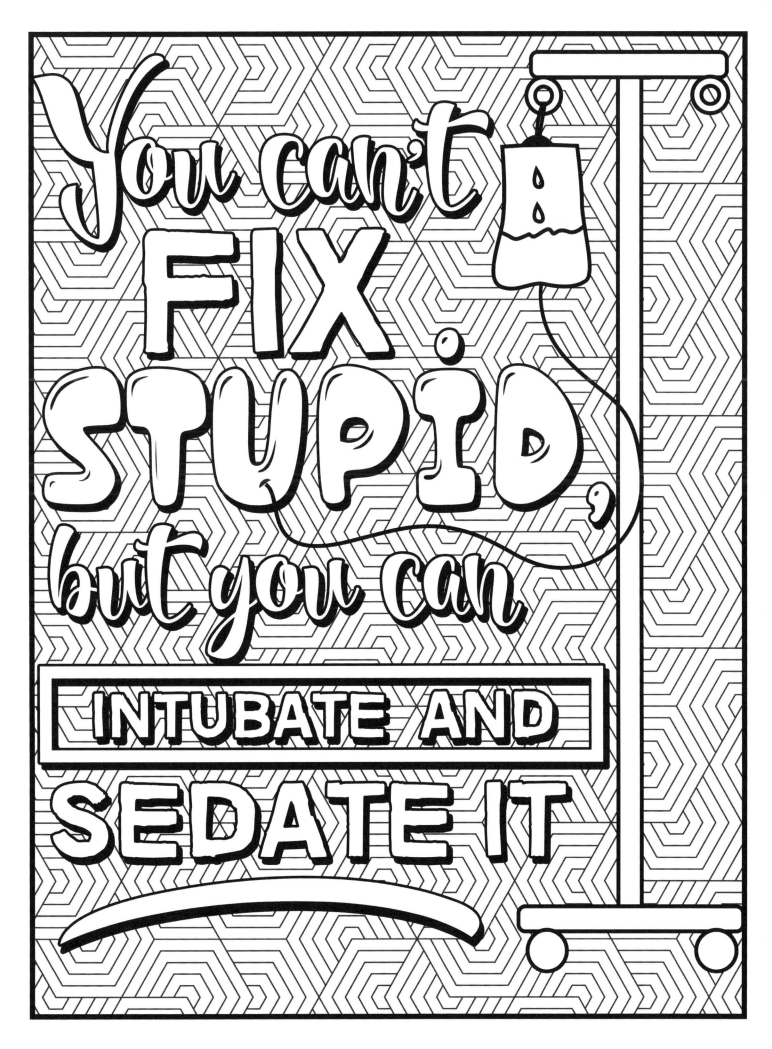

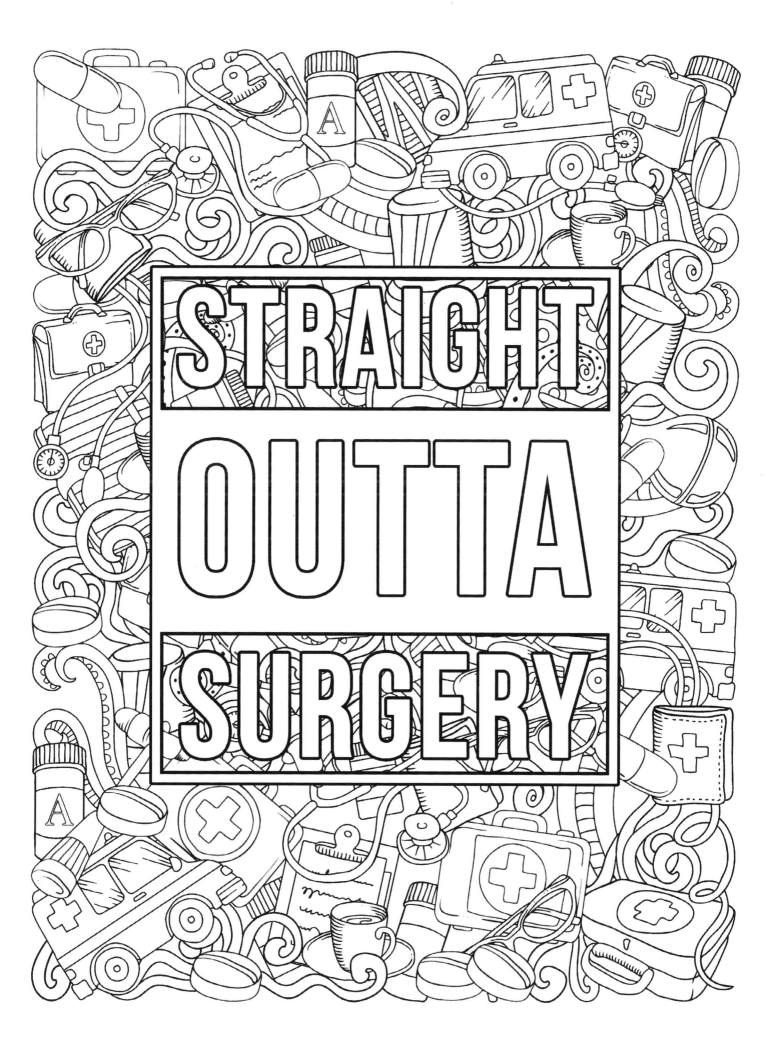

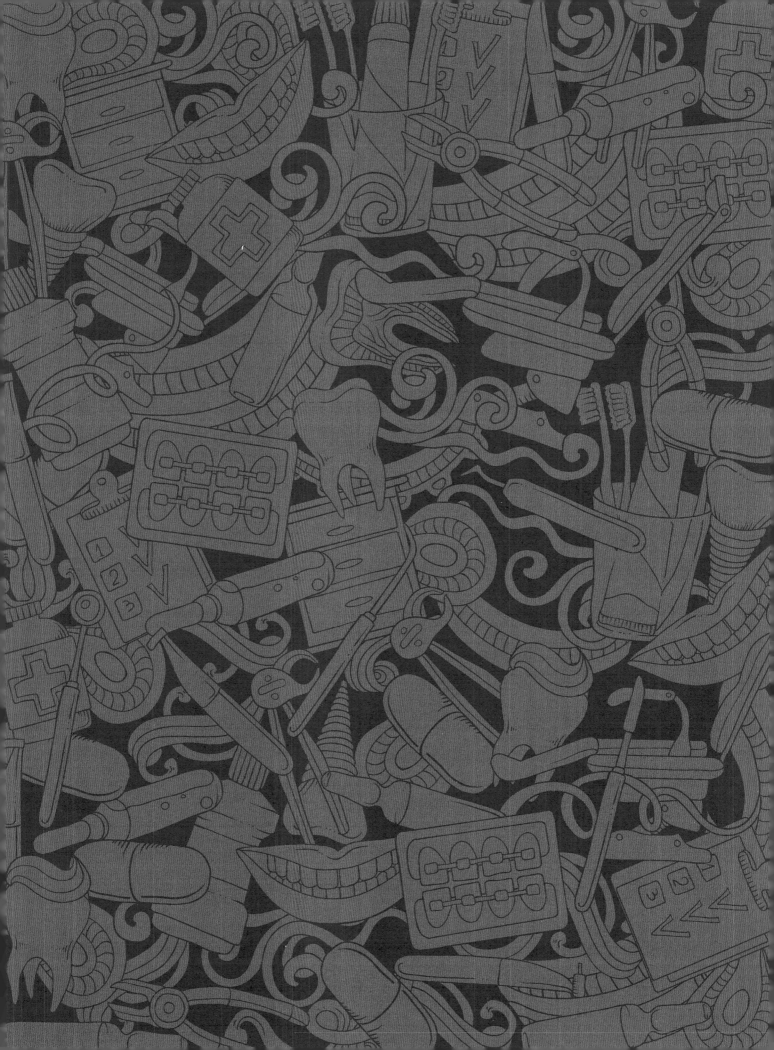

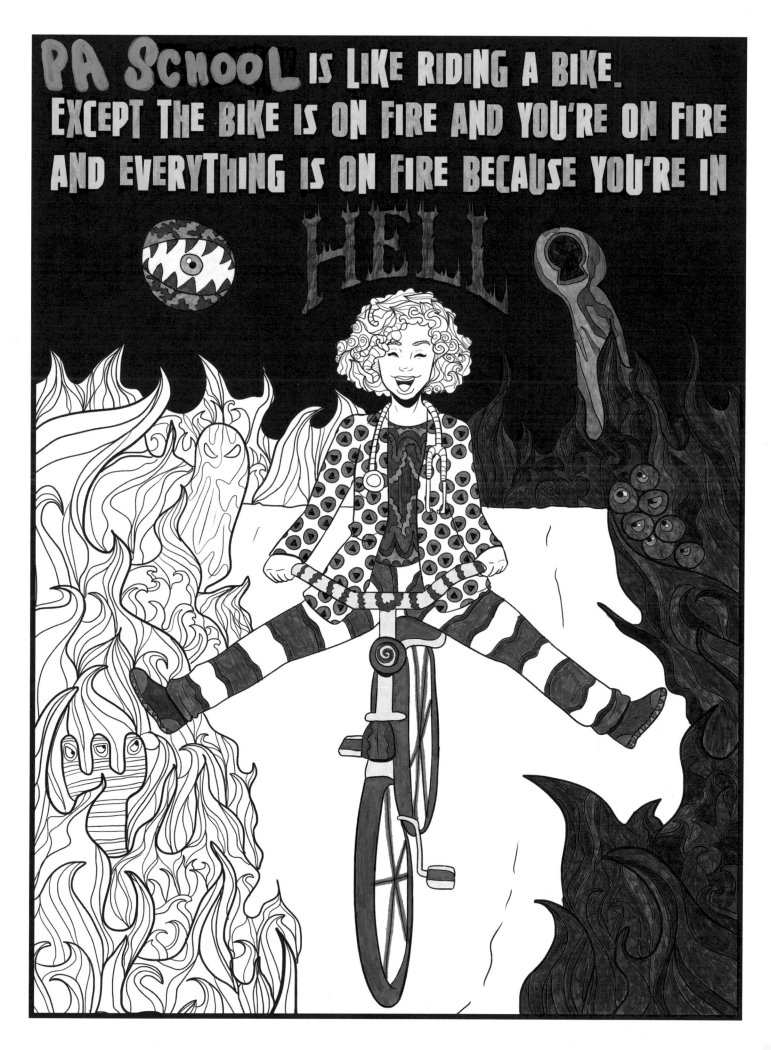

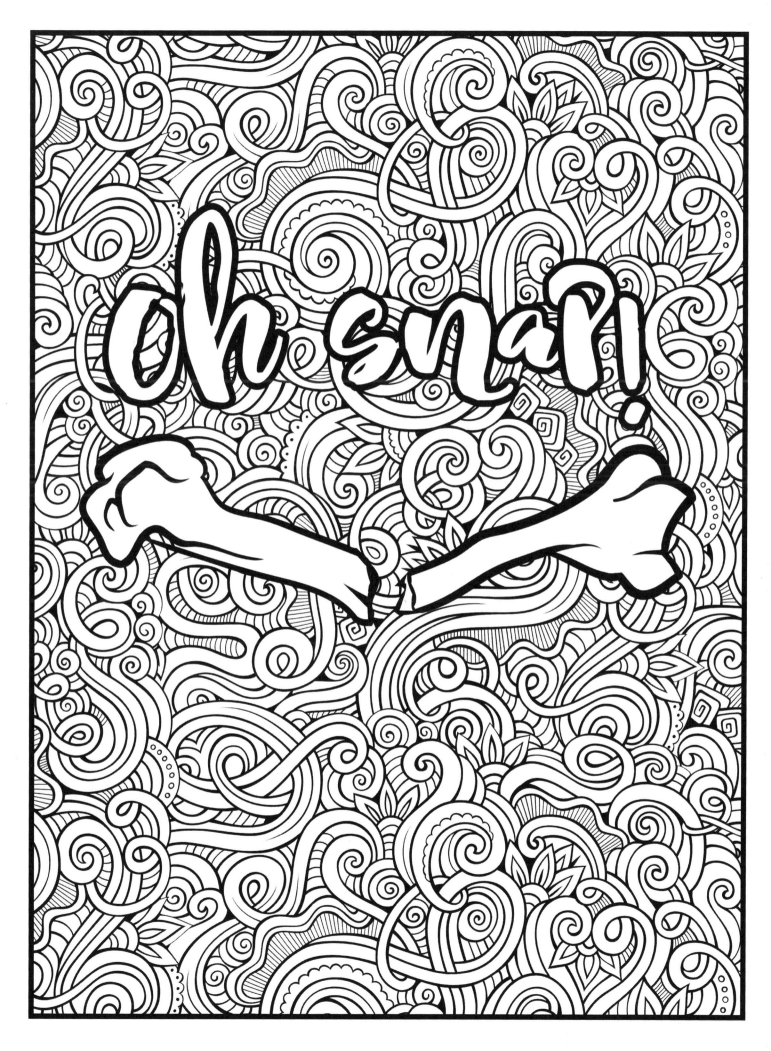

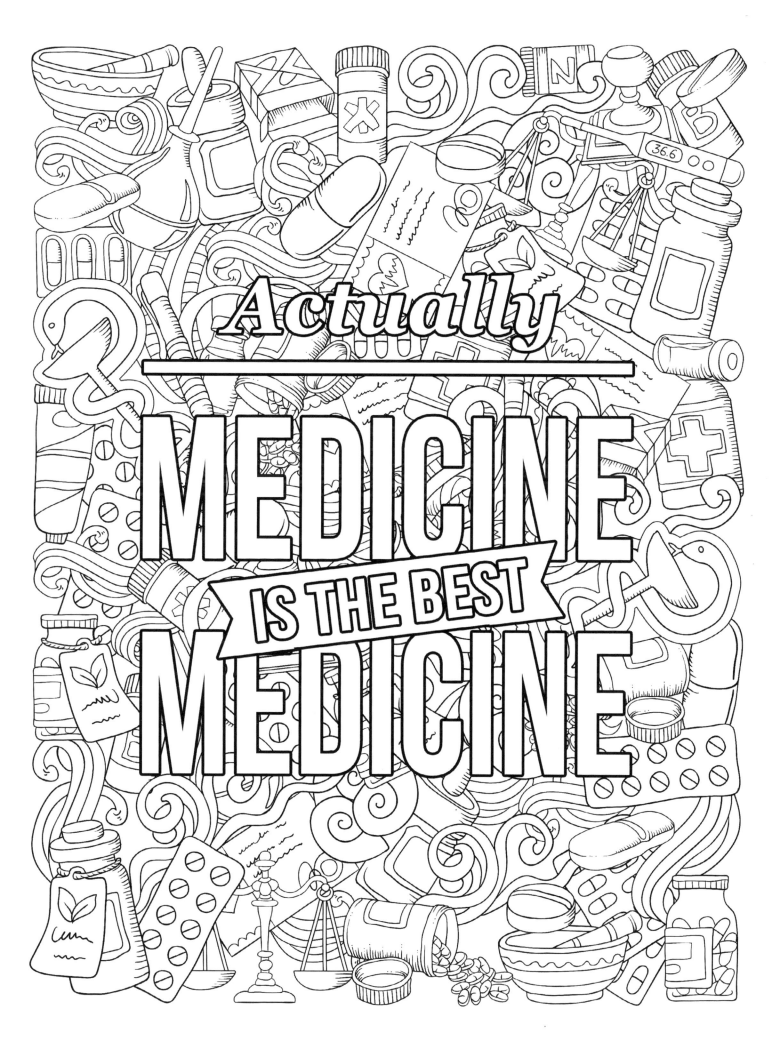

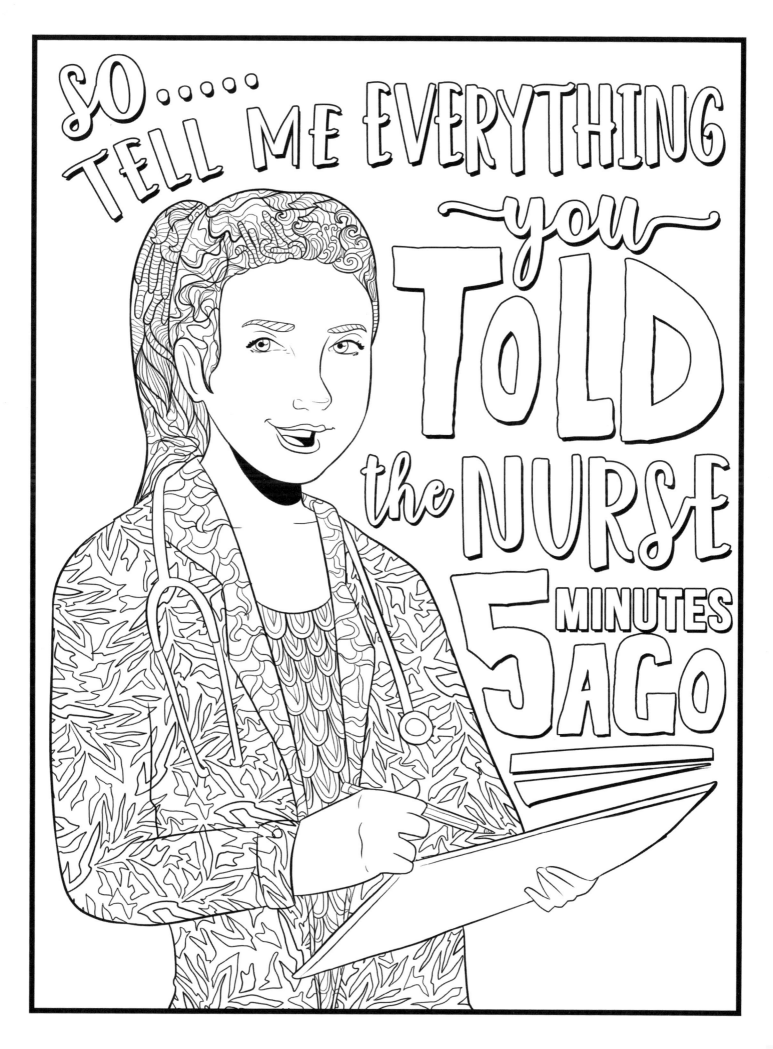

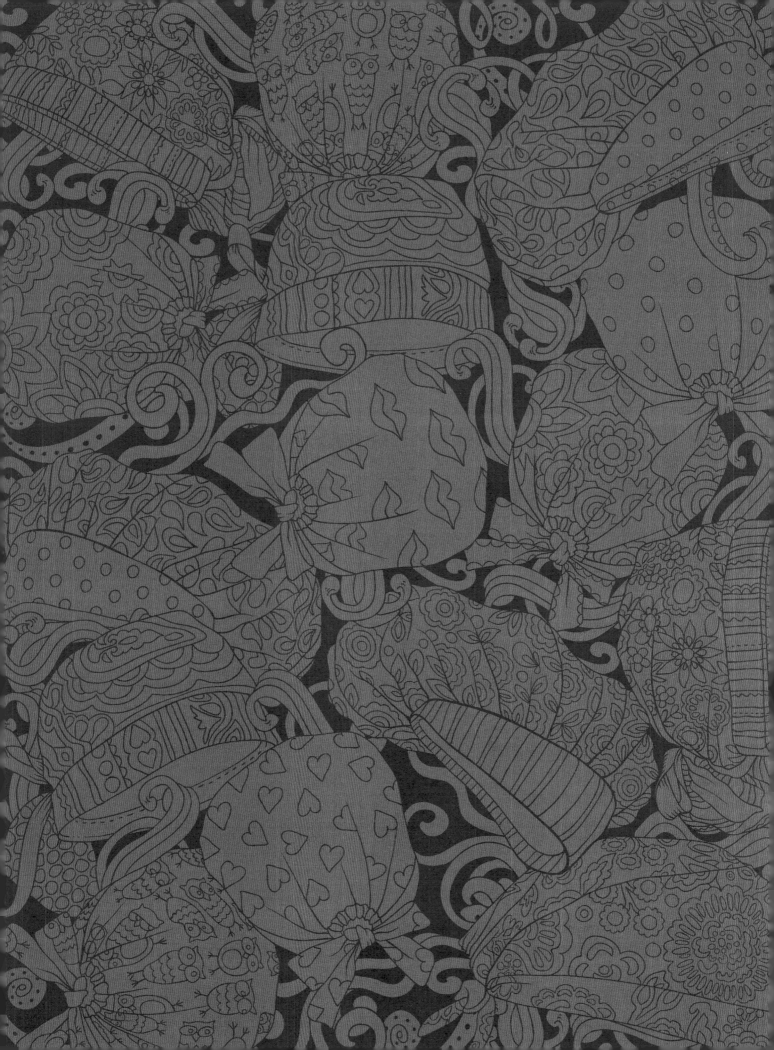

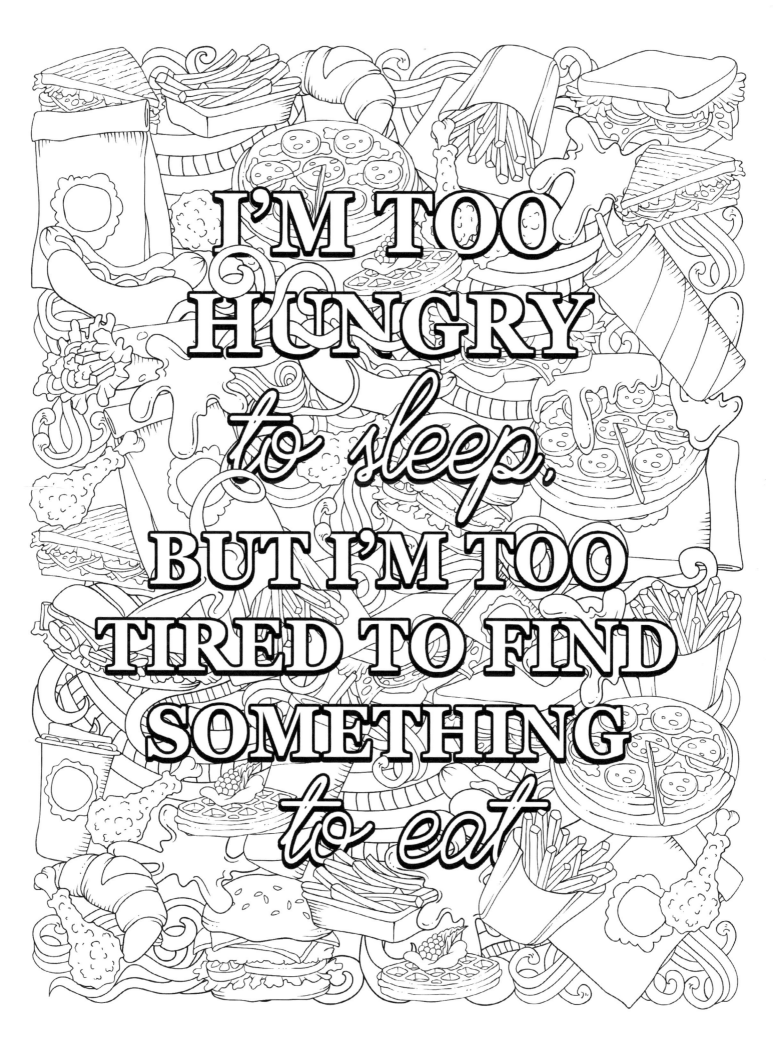

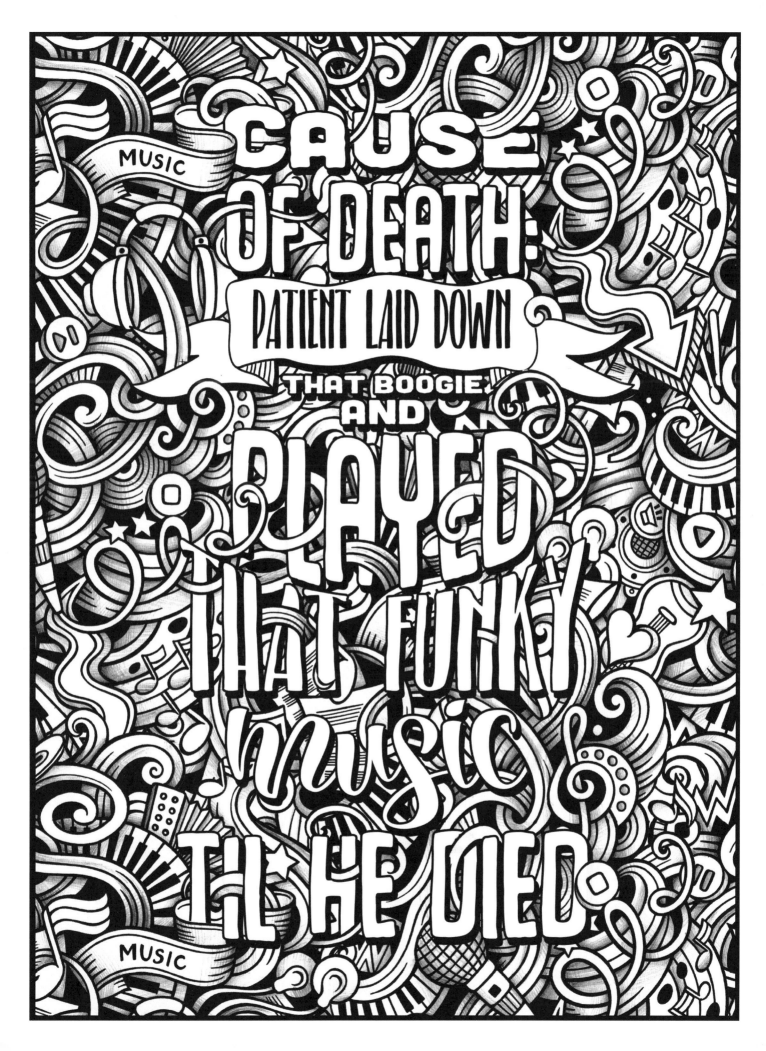

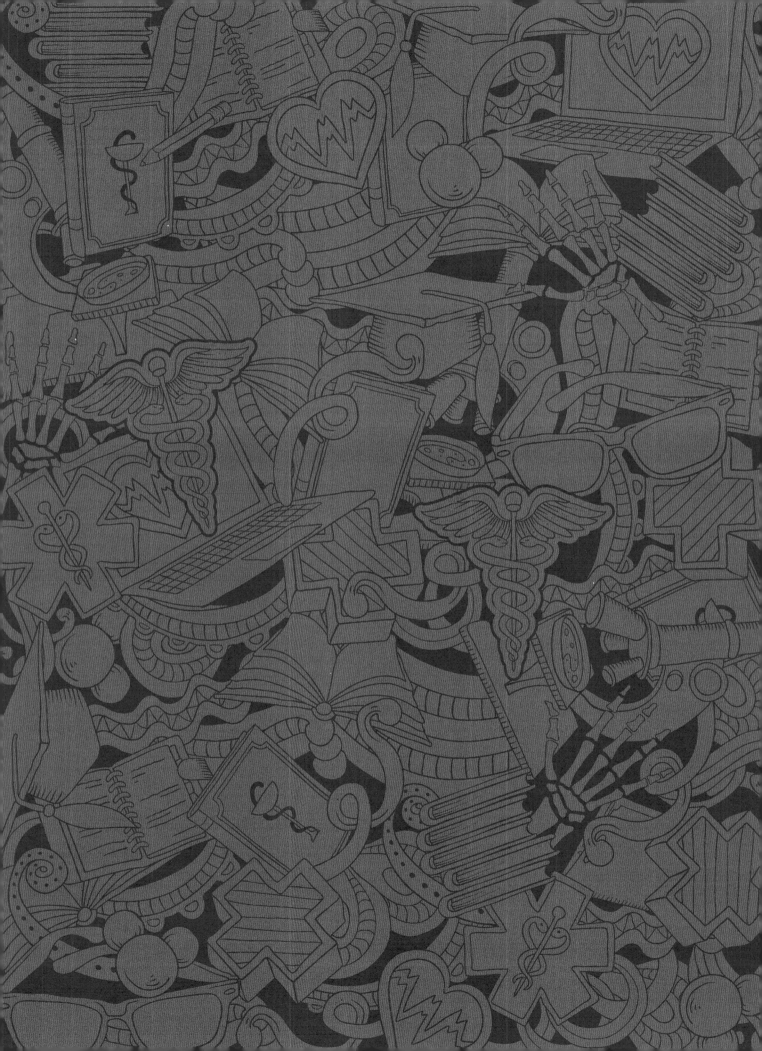

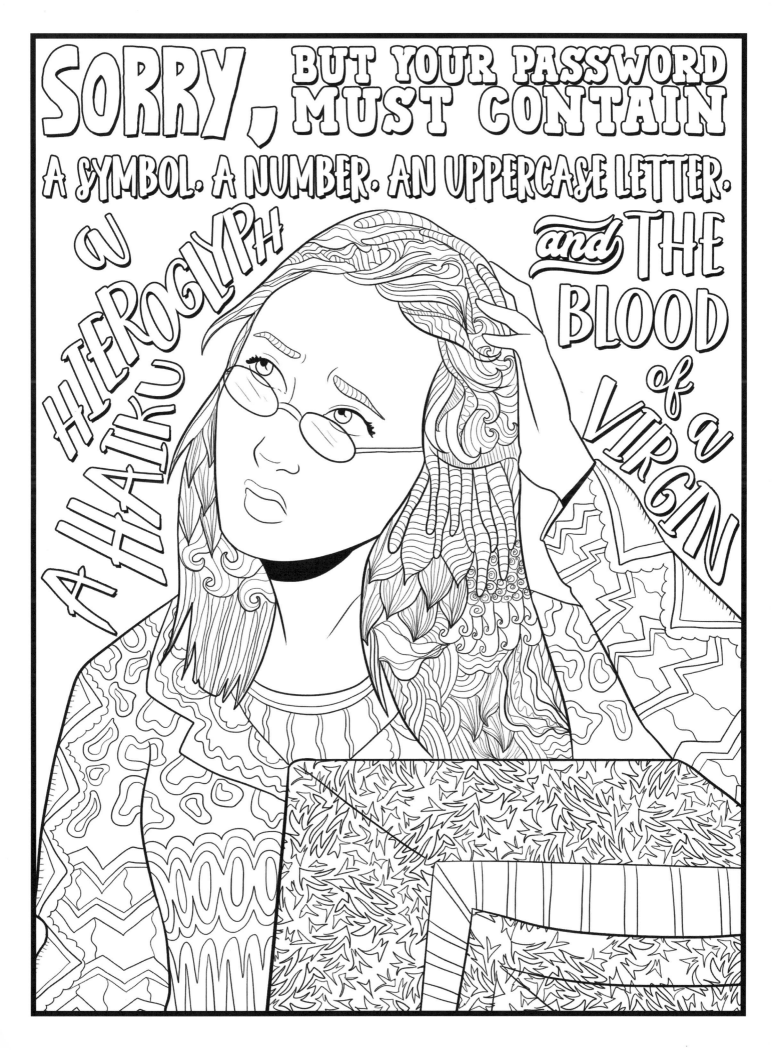

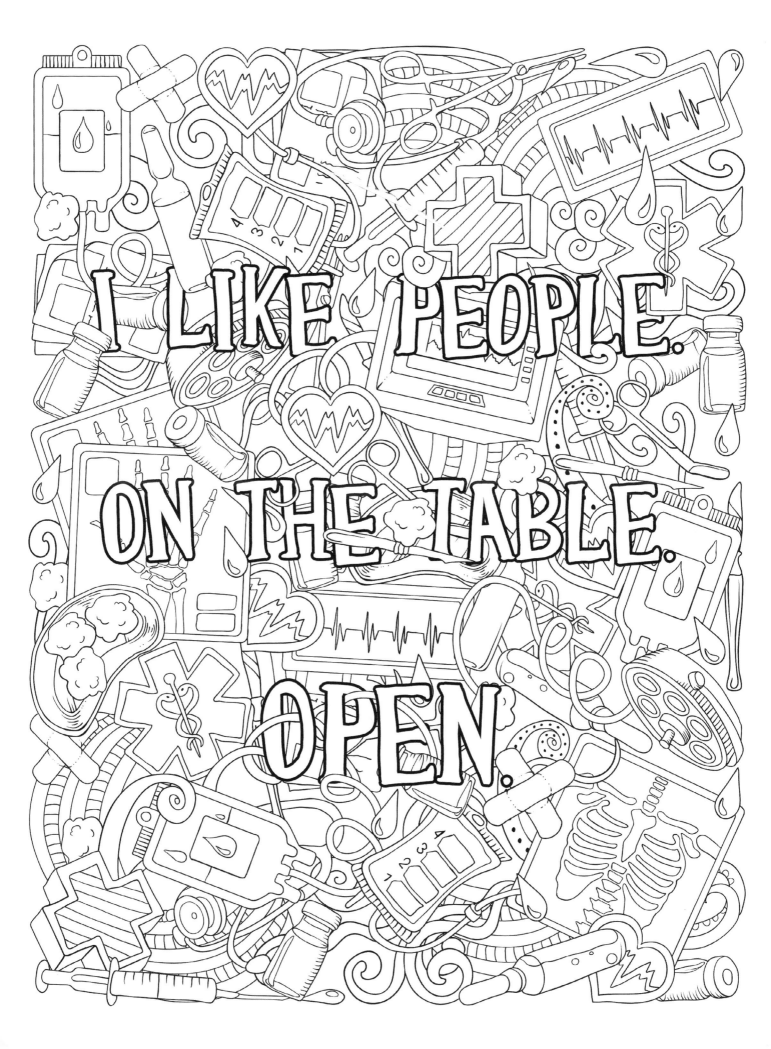

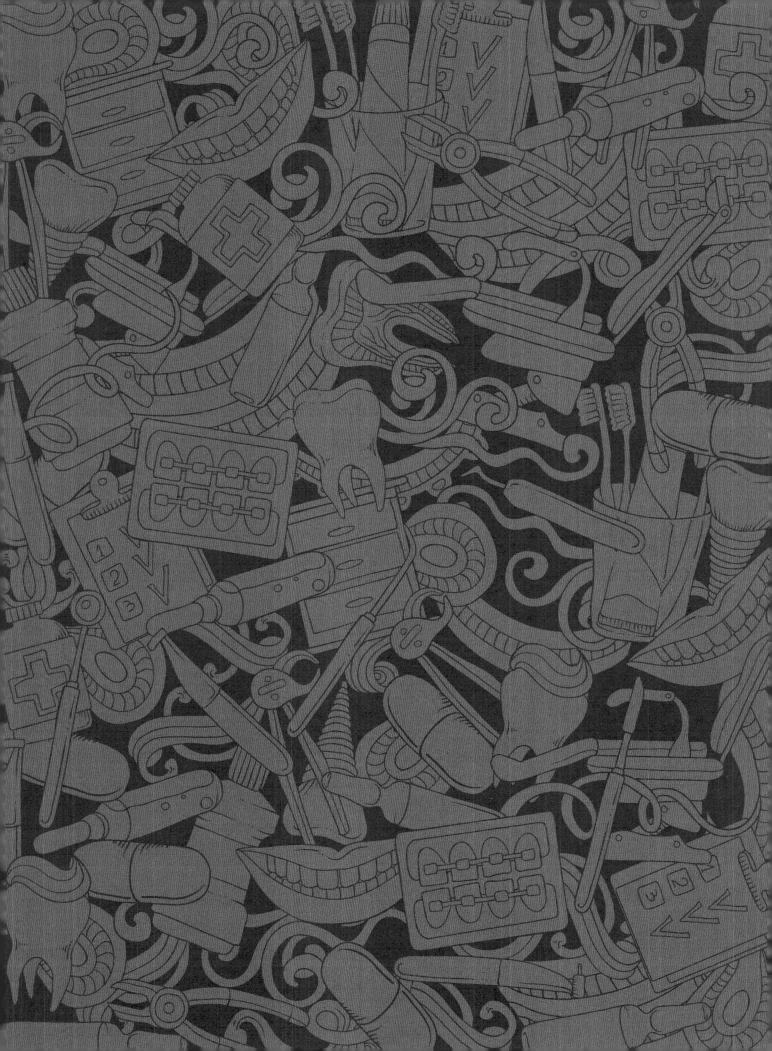

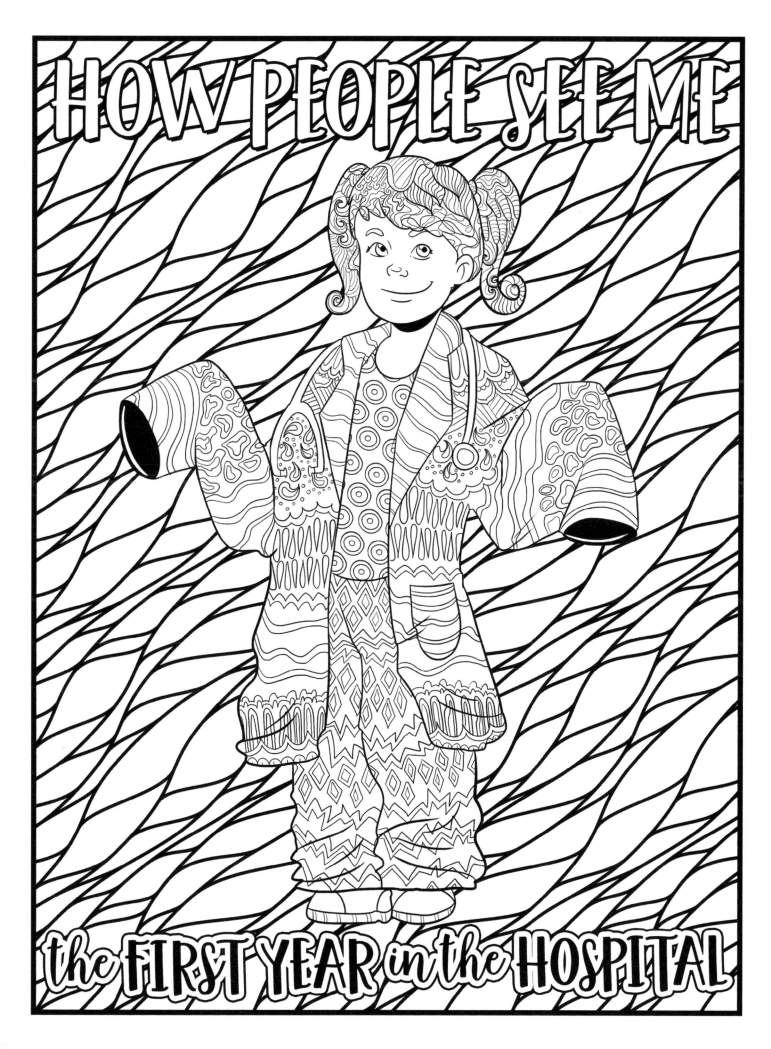

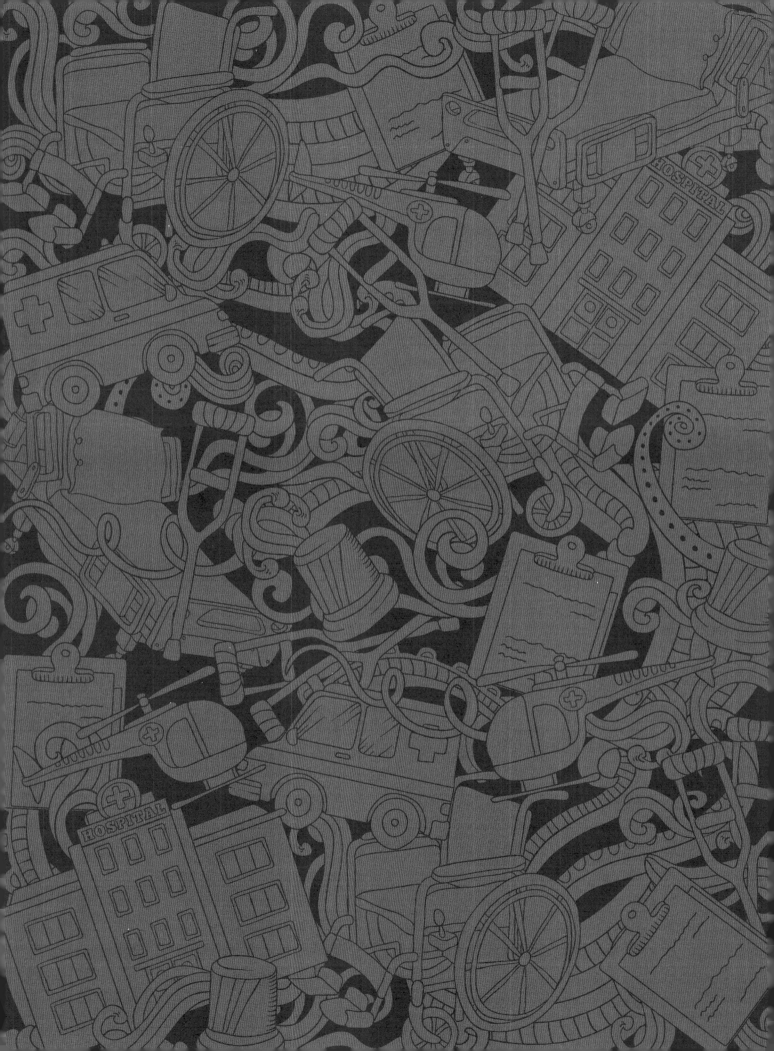

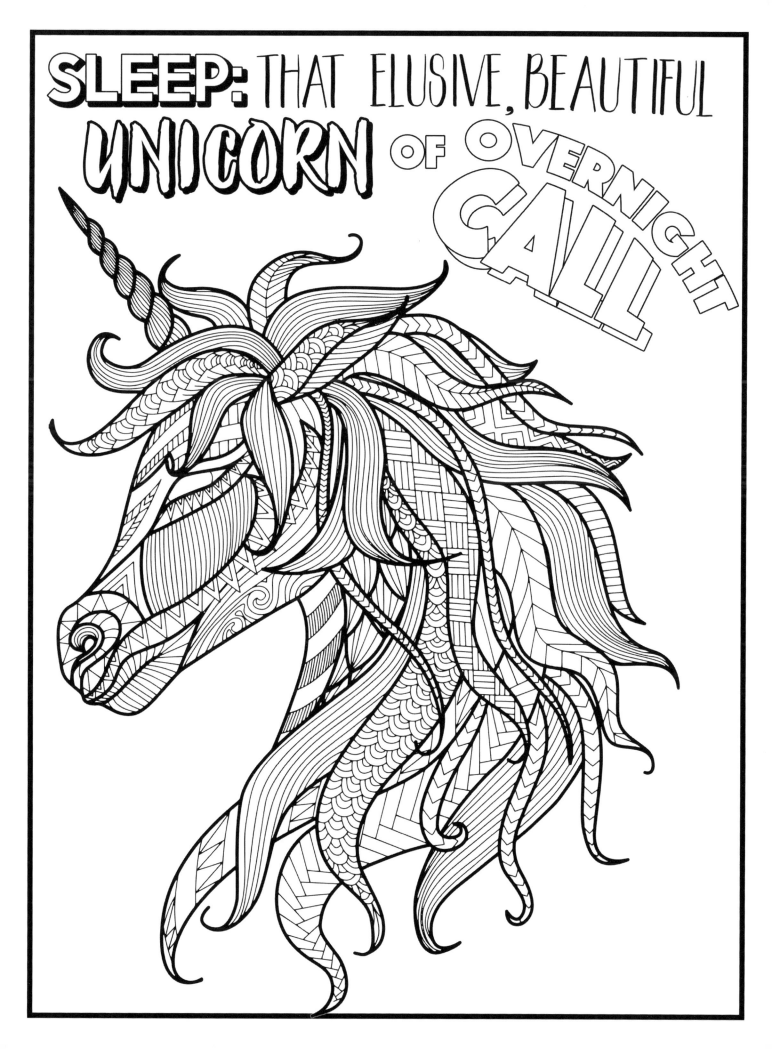

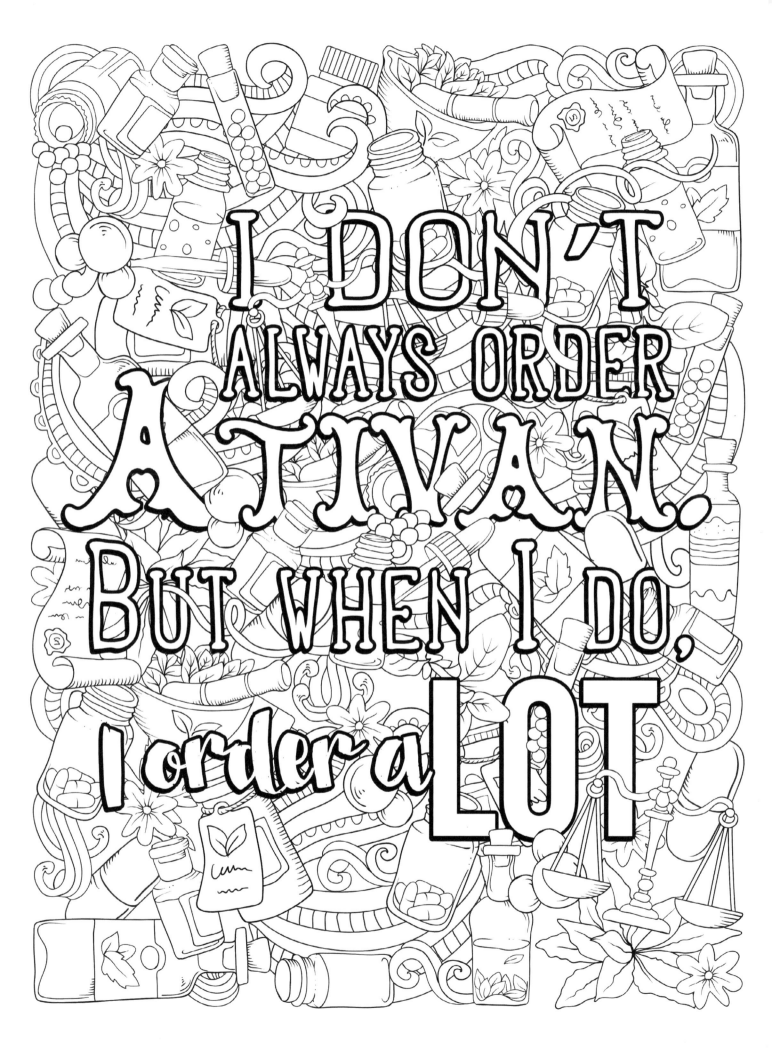

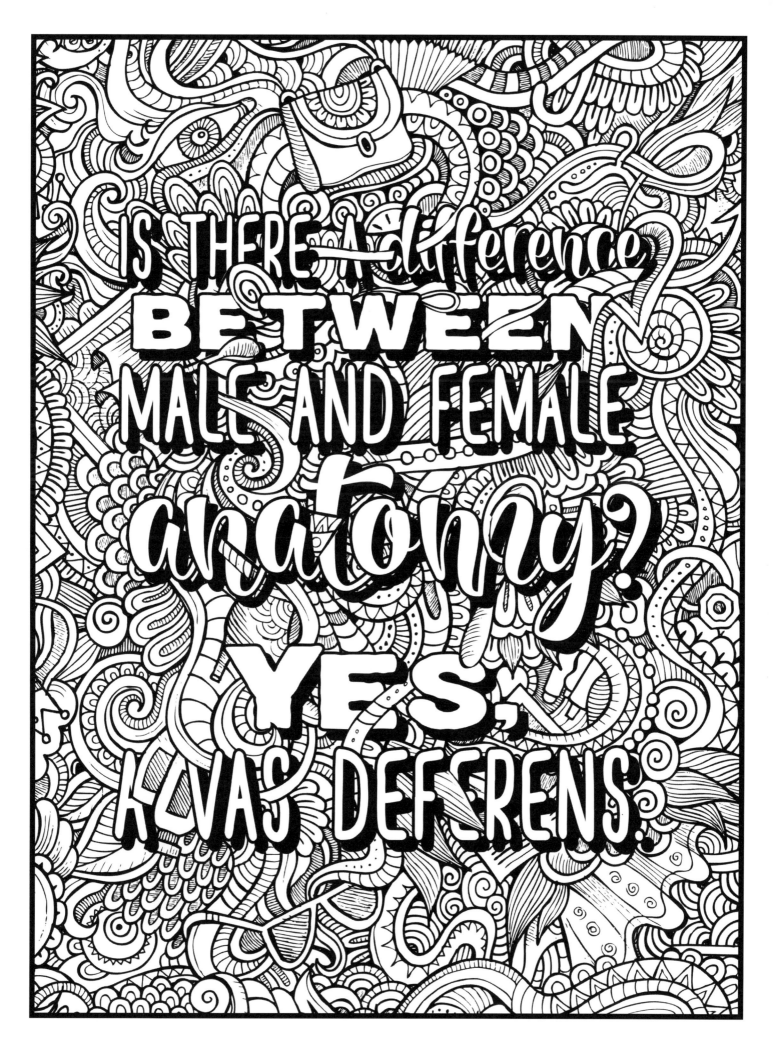

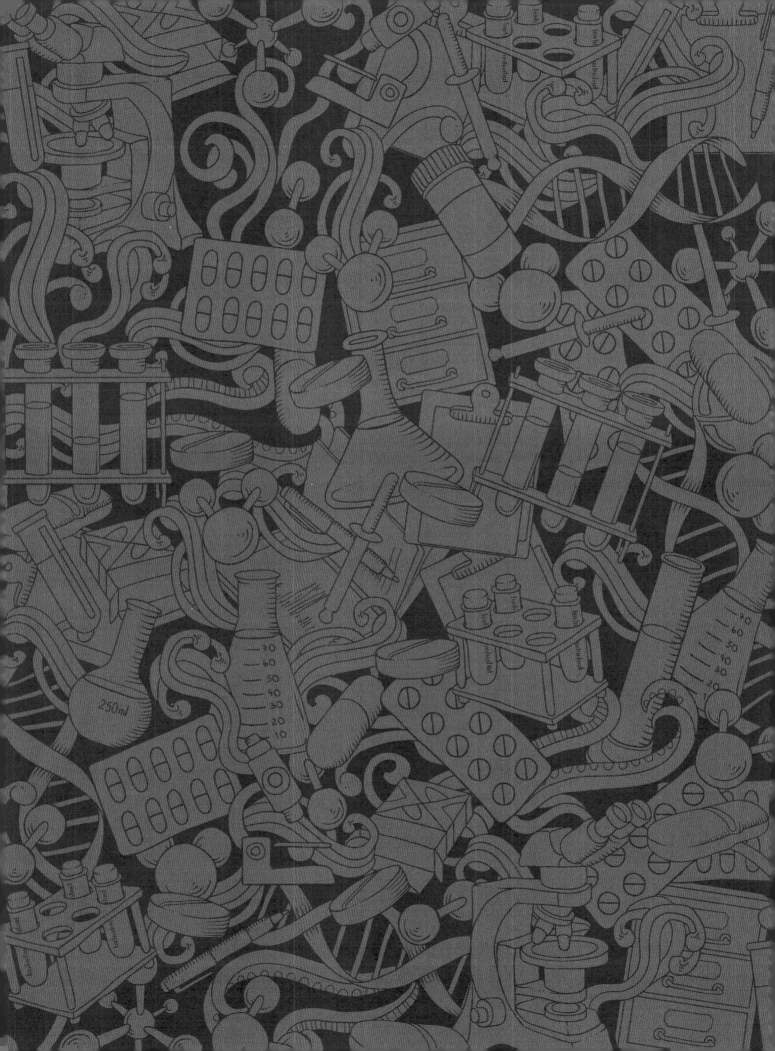

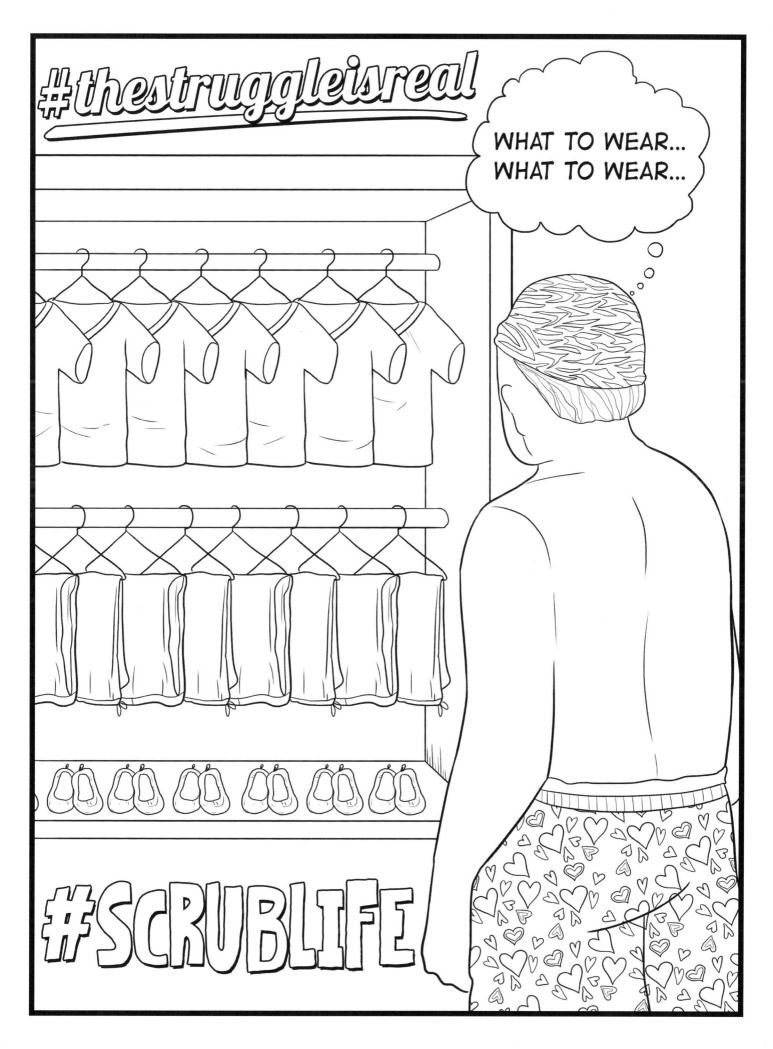

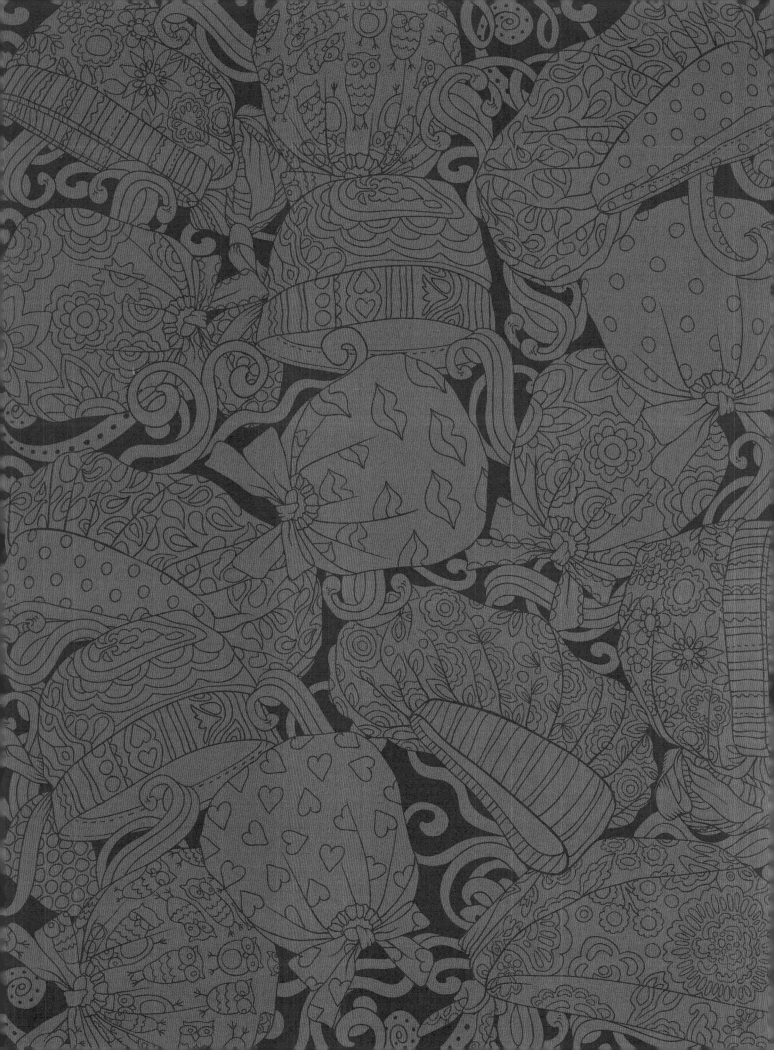

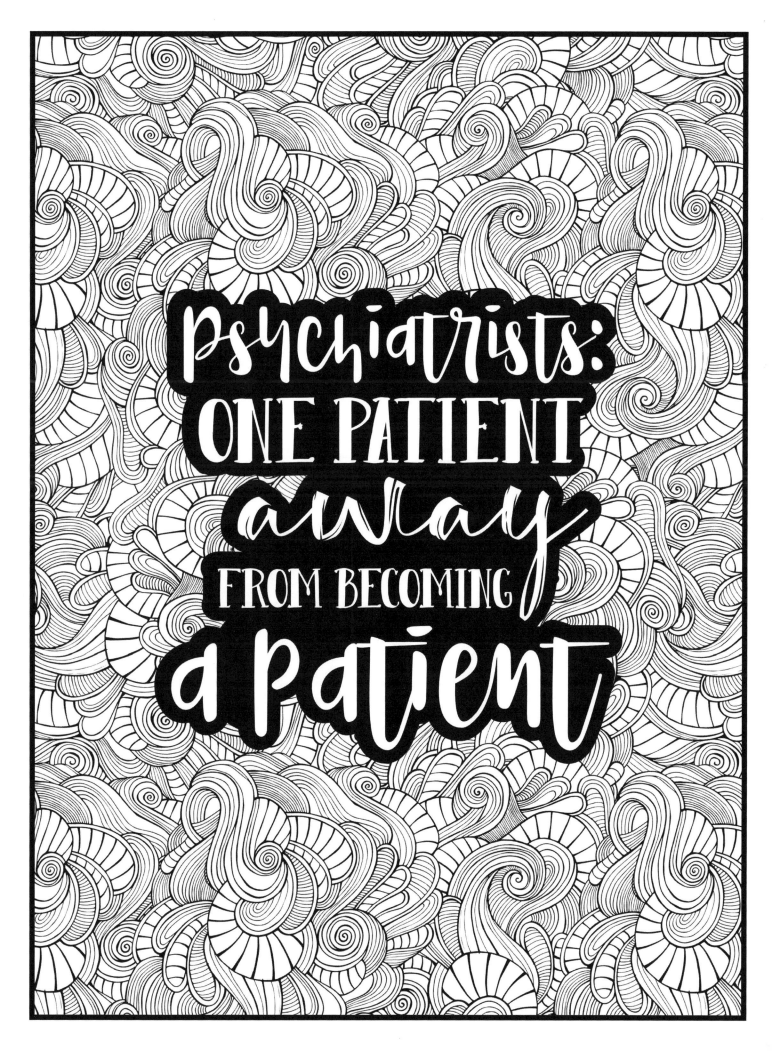

Psychiatrists: ONE PATIENT away FROM BECOMING a patient

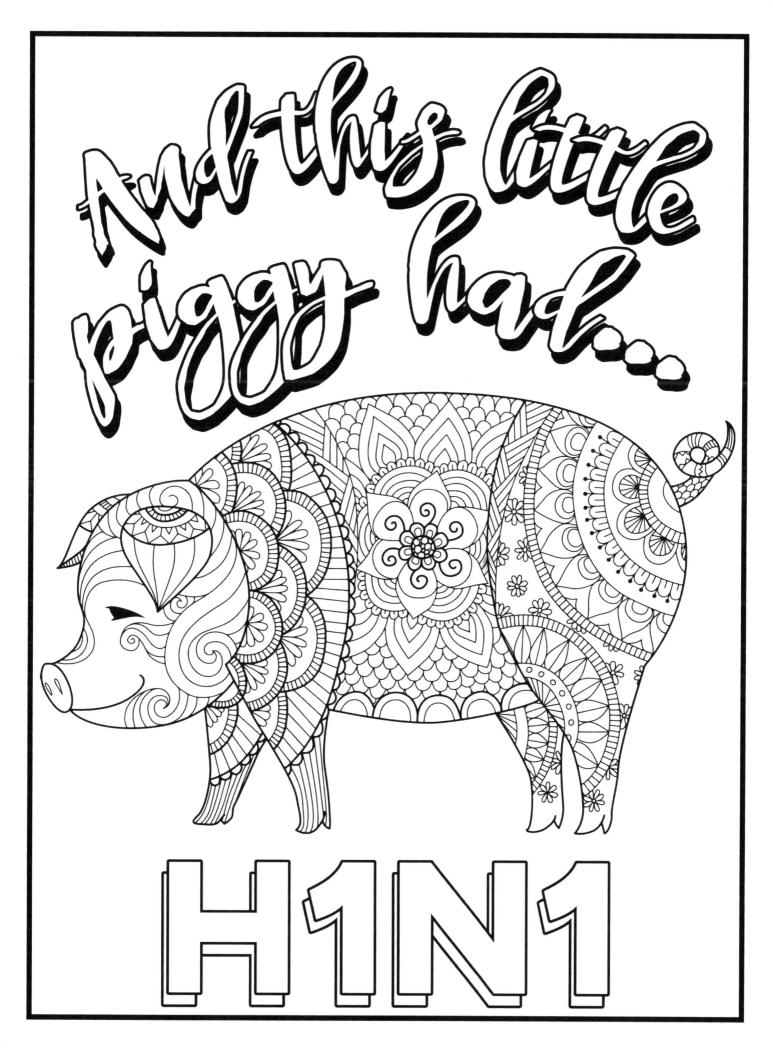

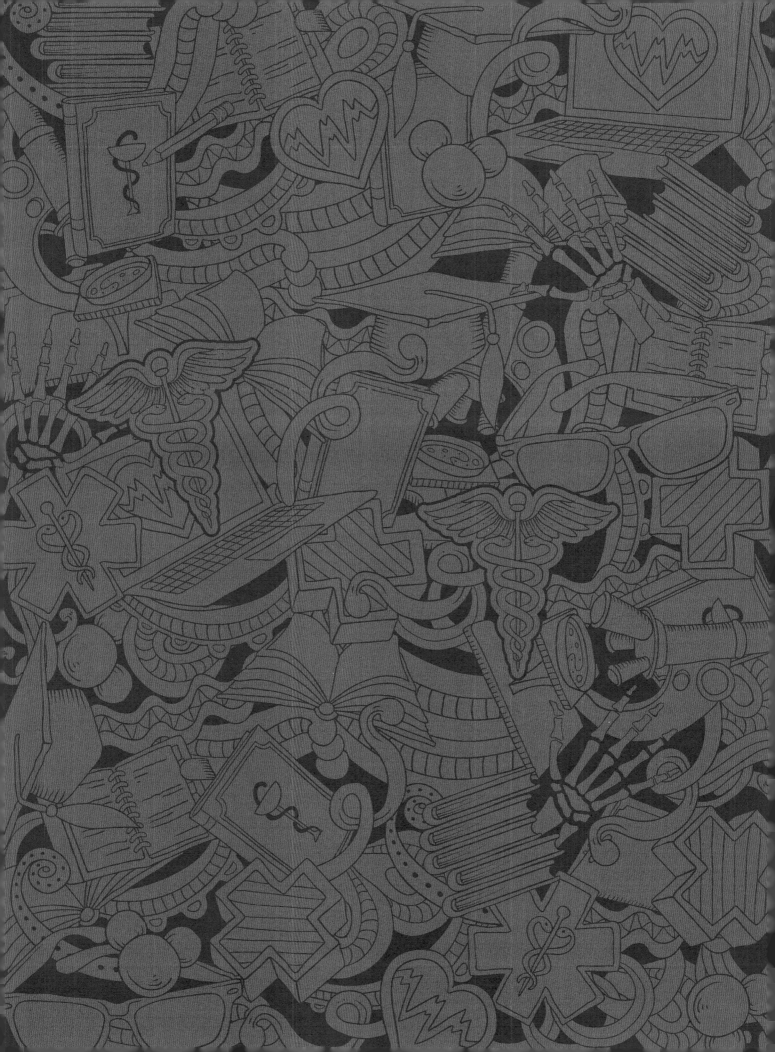

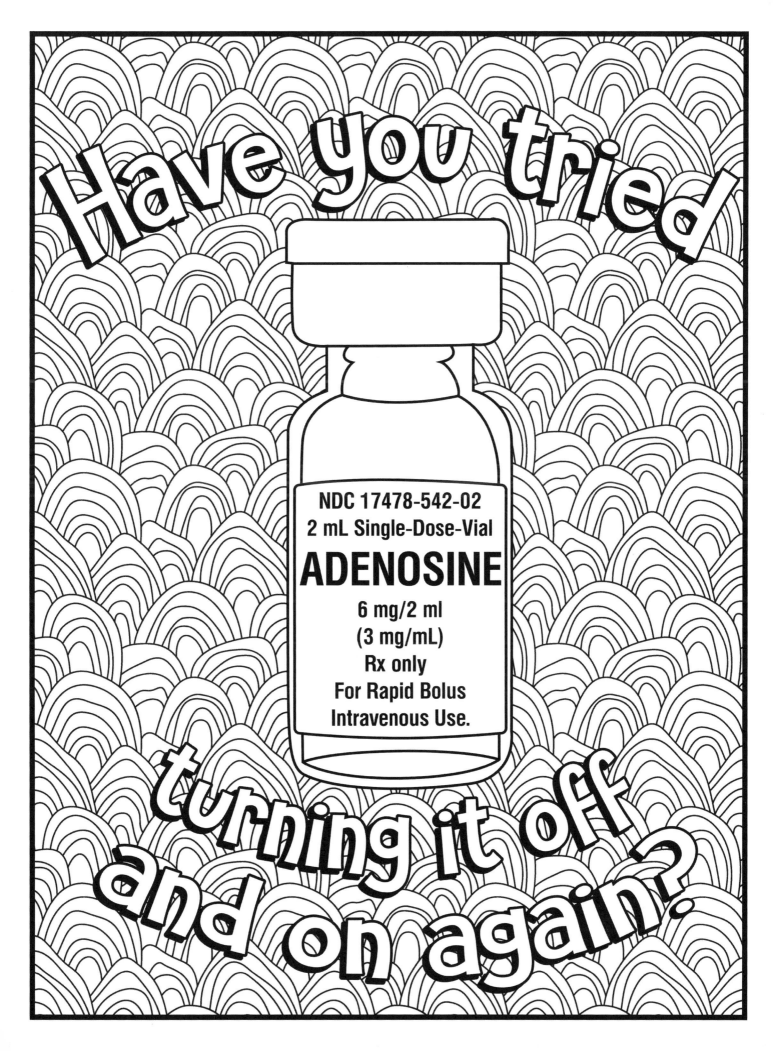

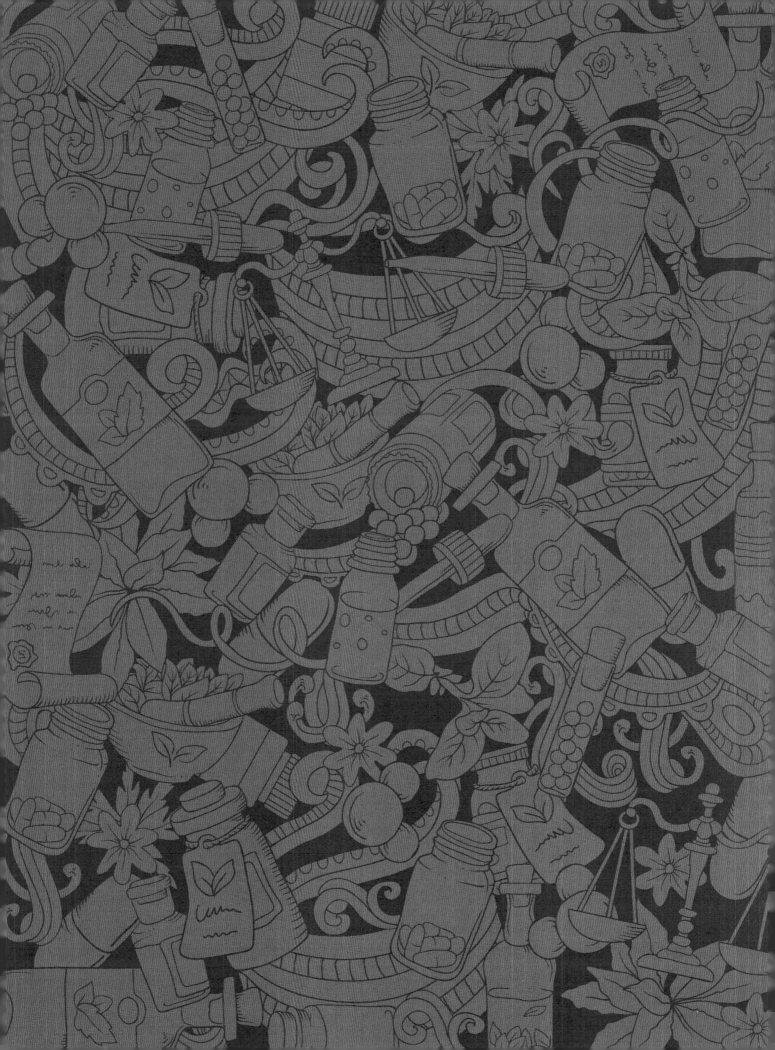

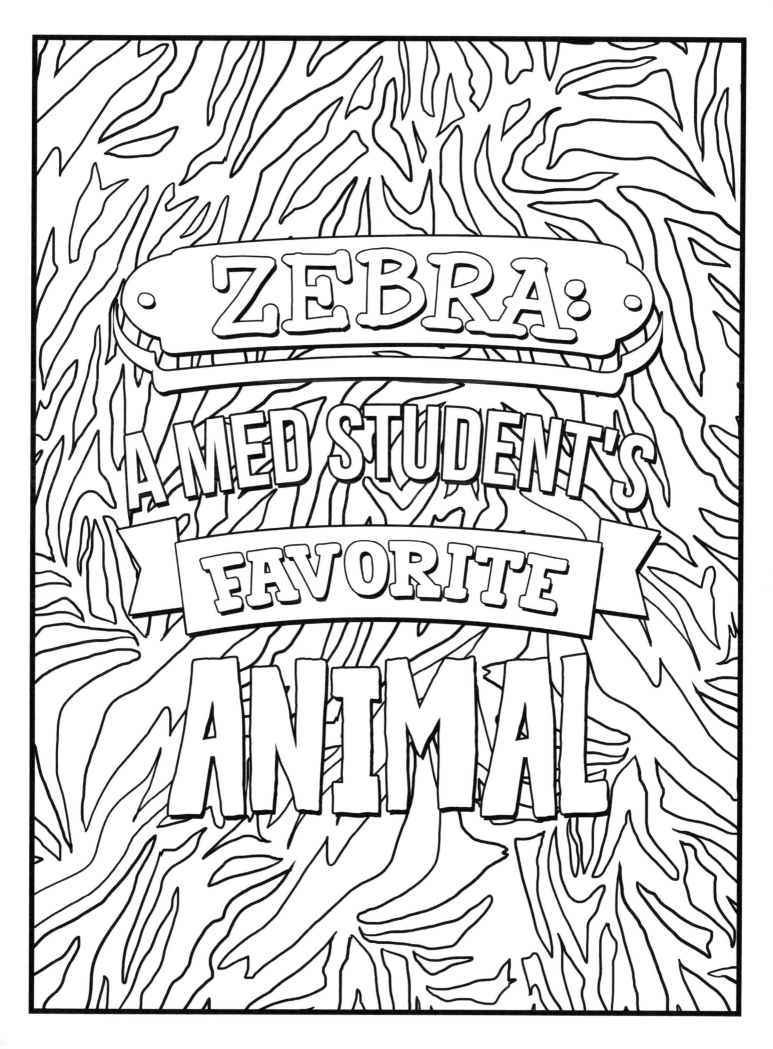

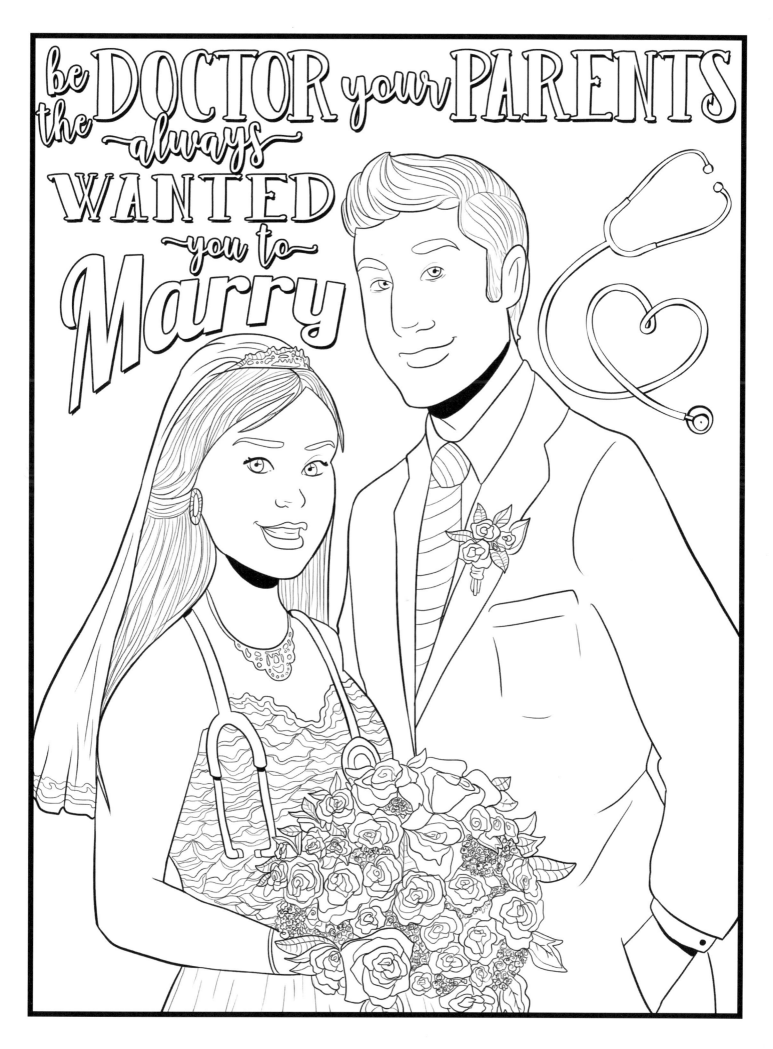

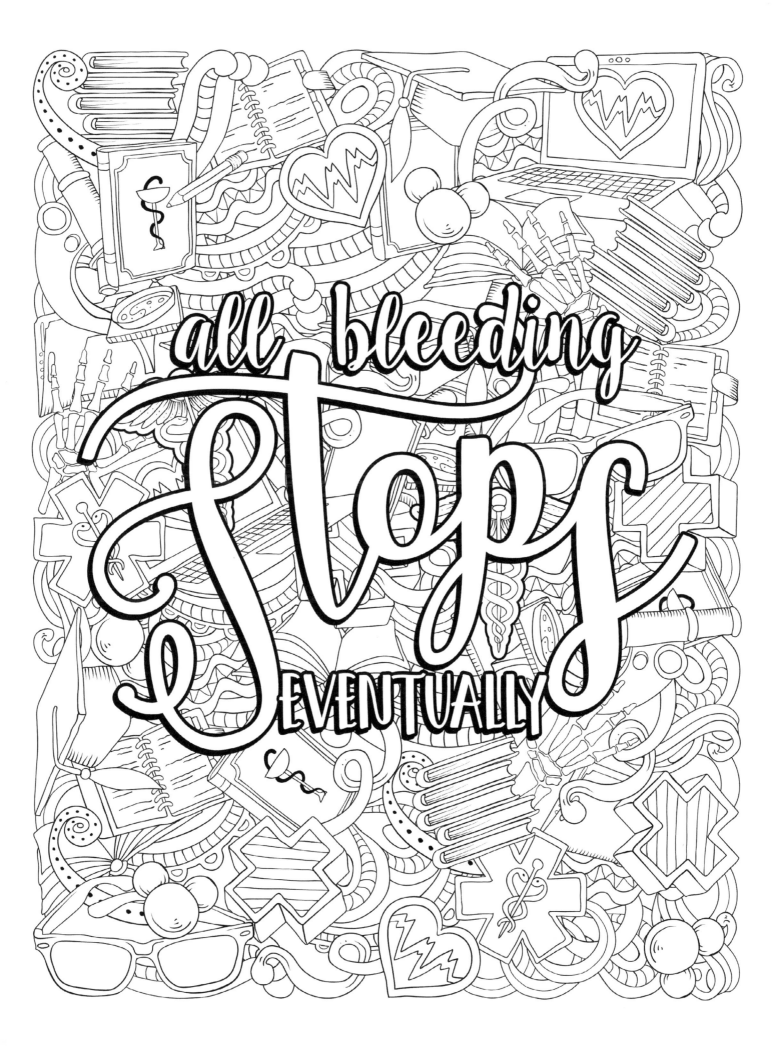

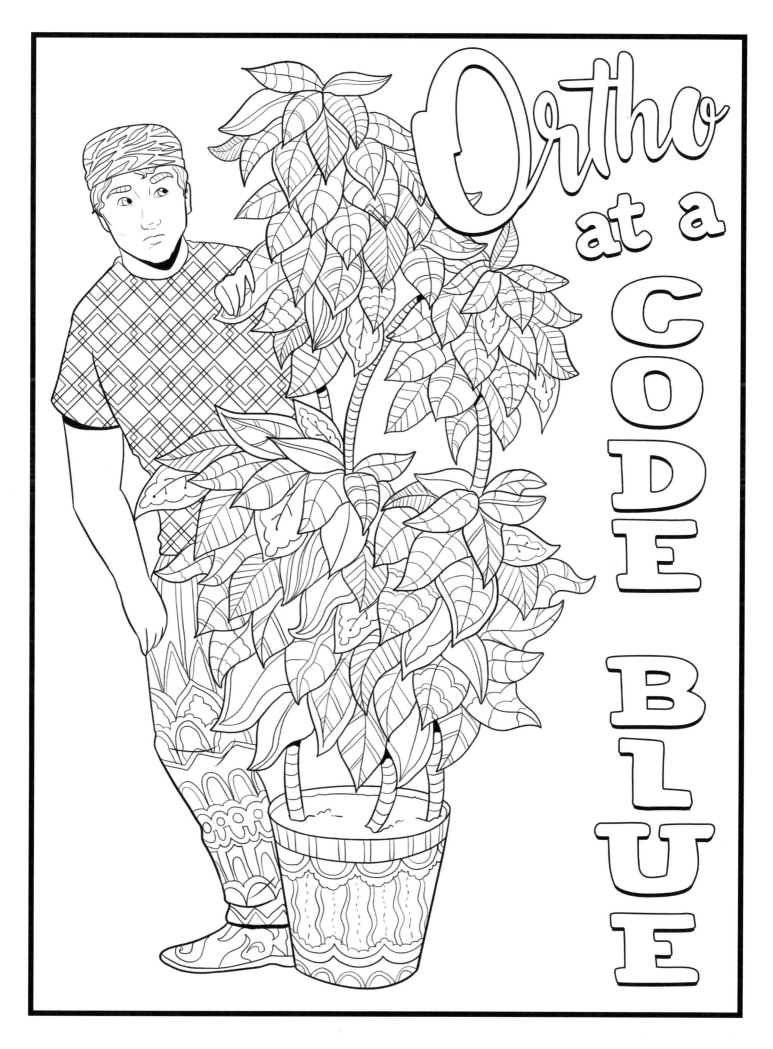

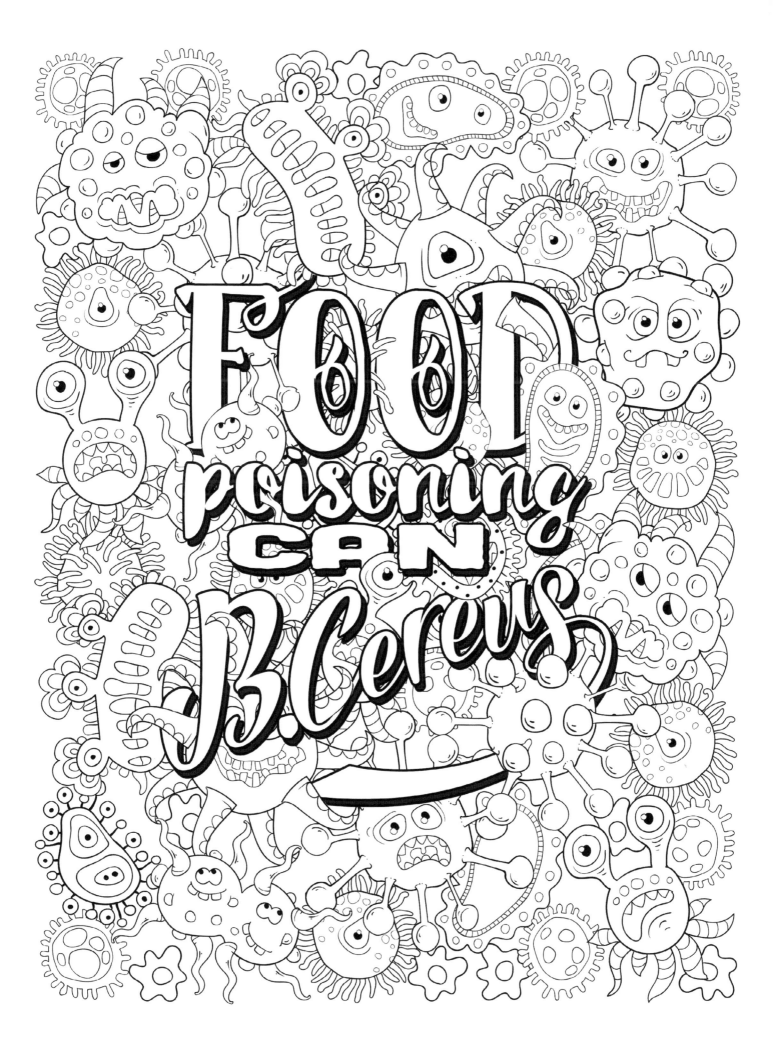

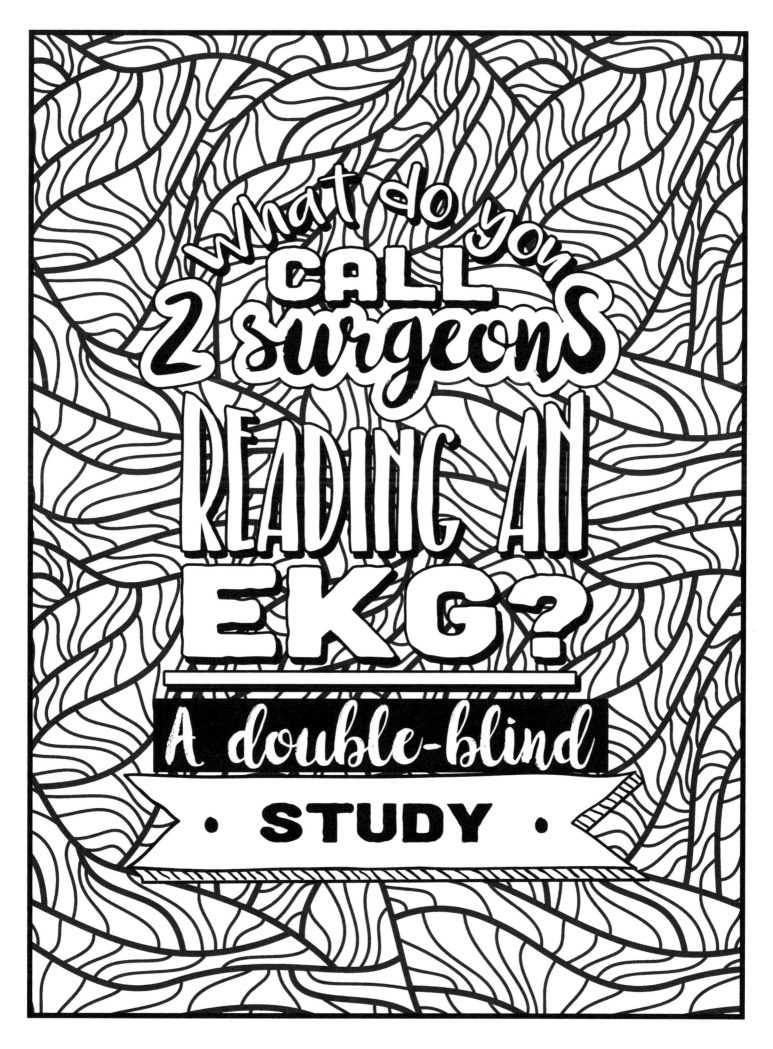

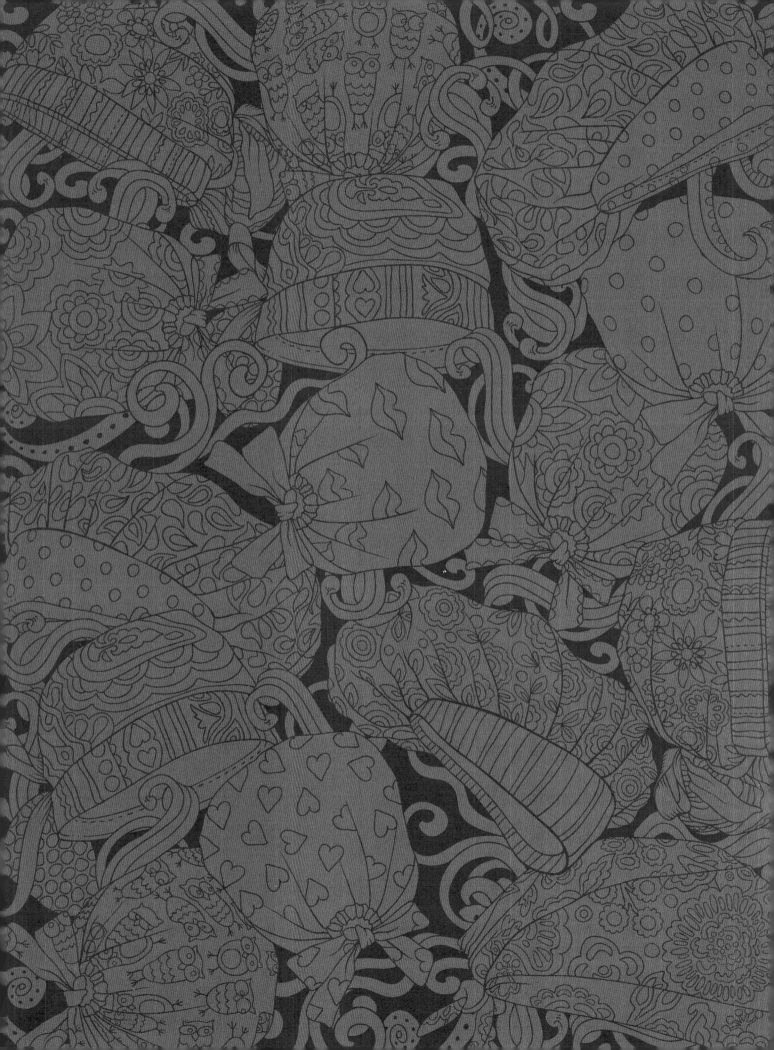

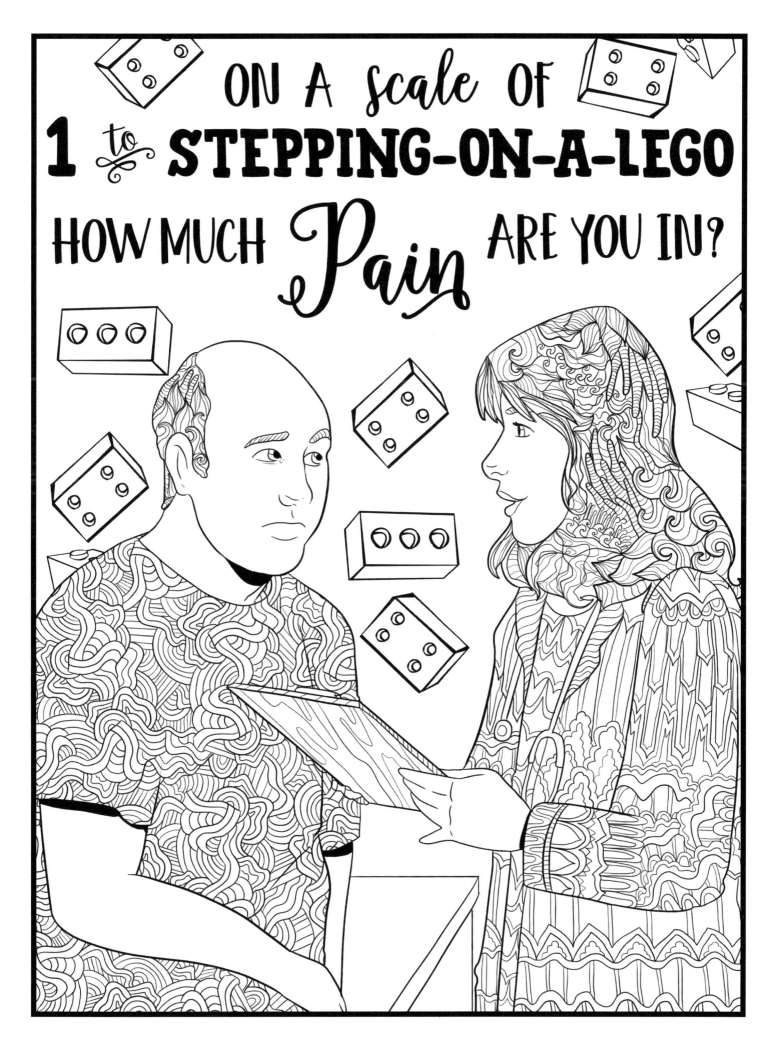

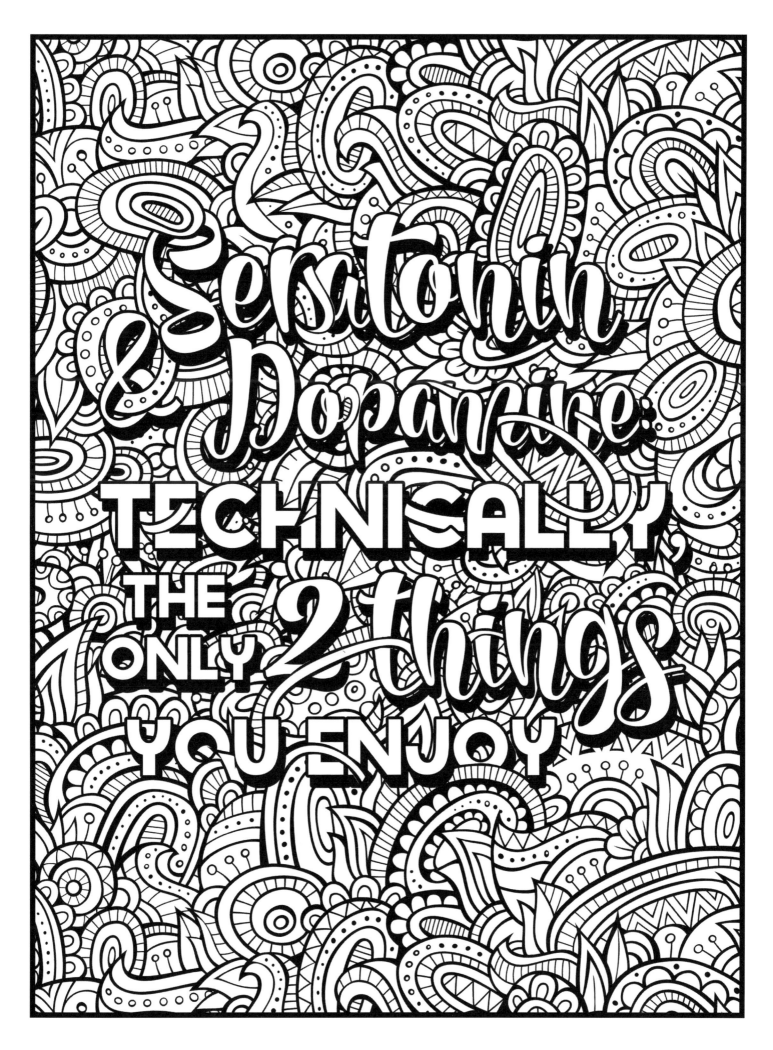

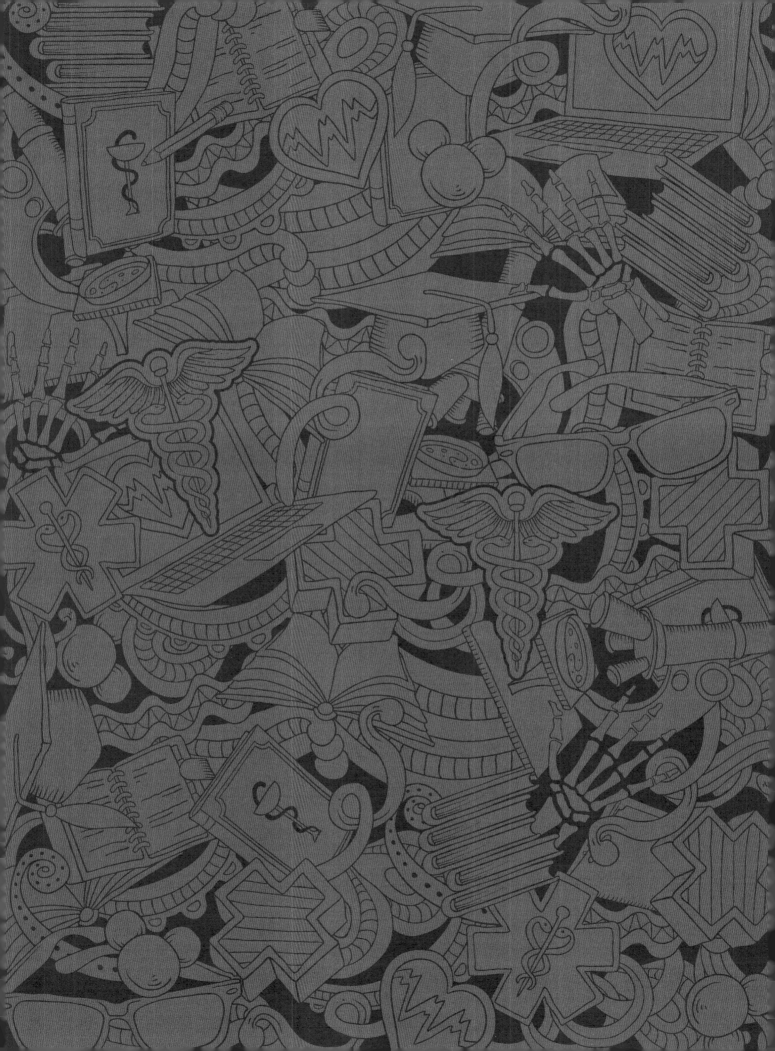

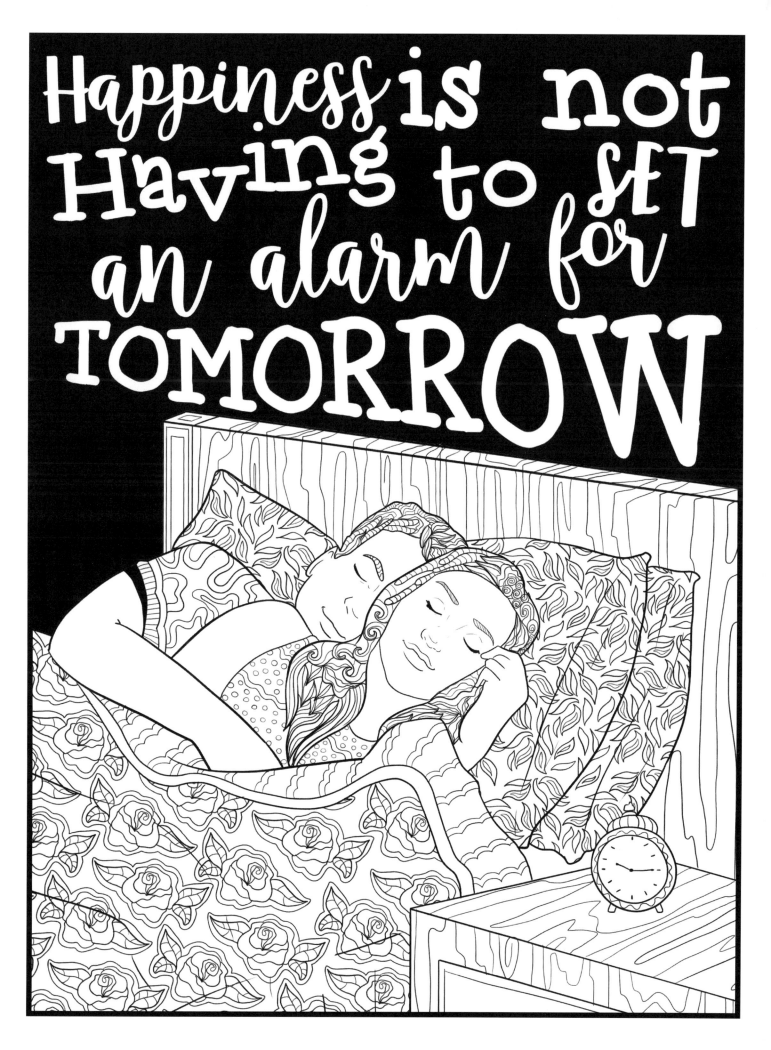

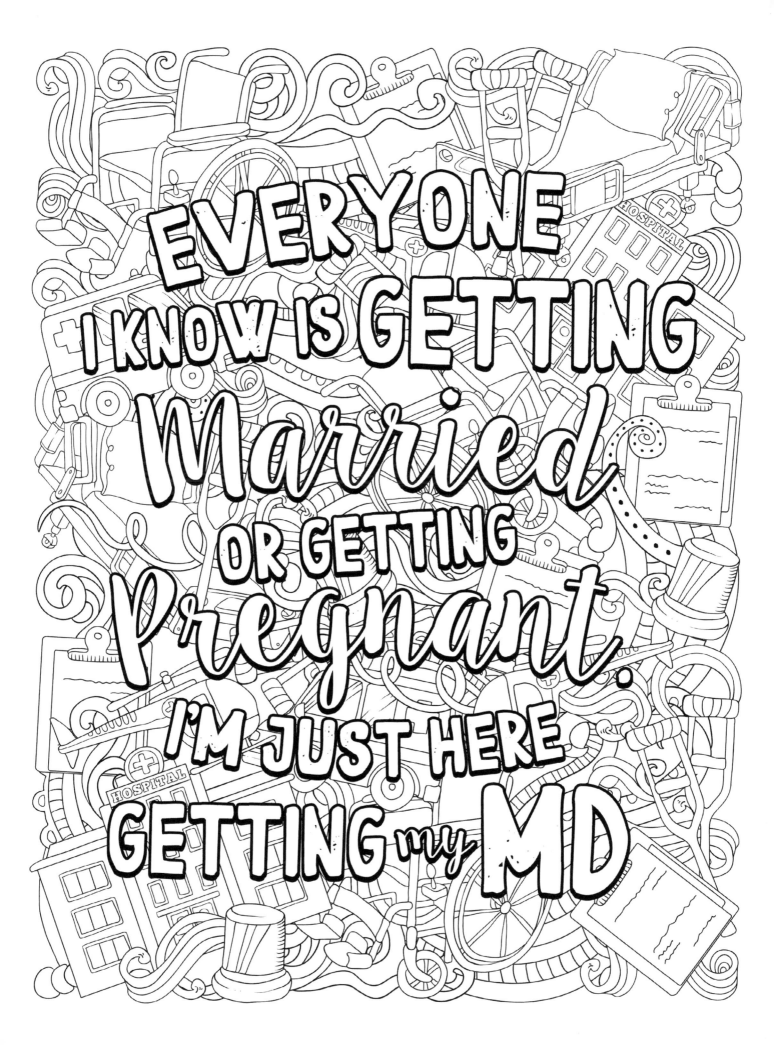

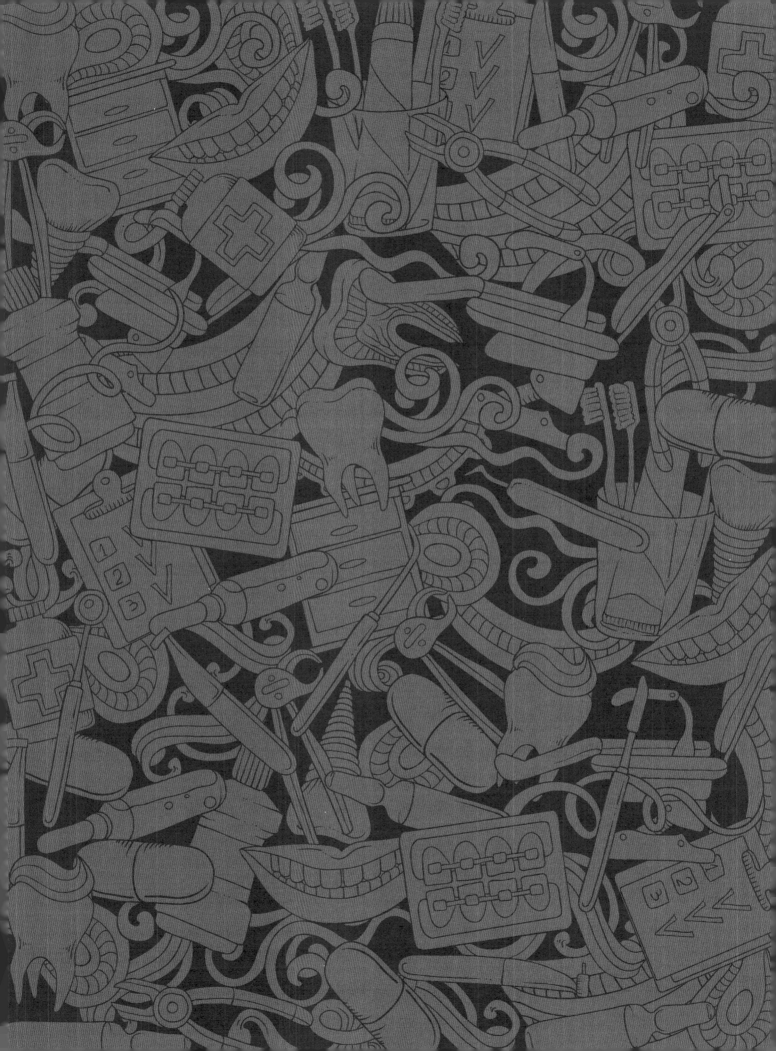

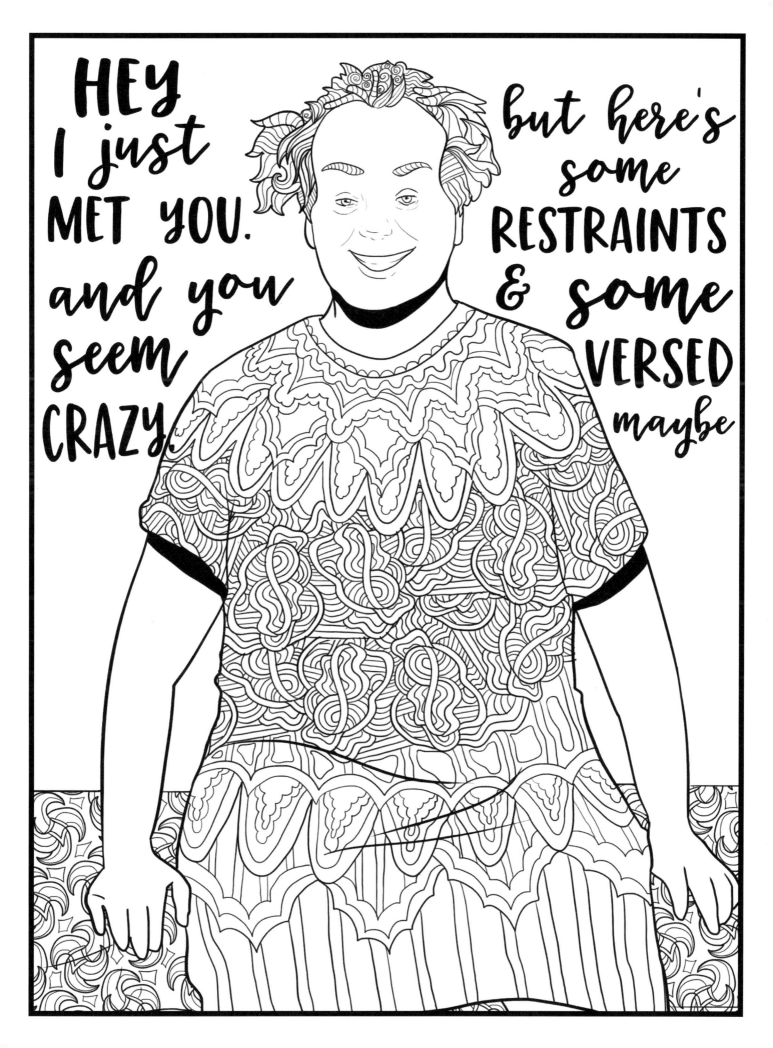

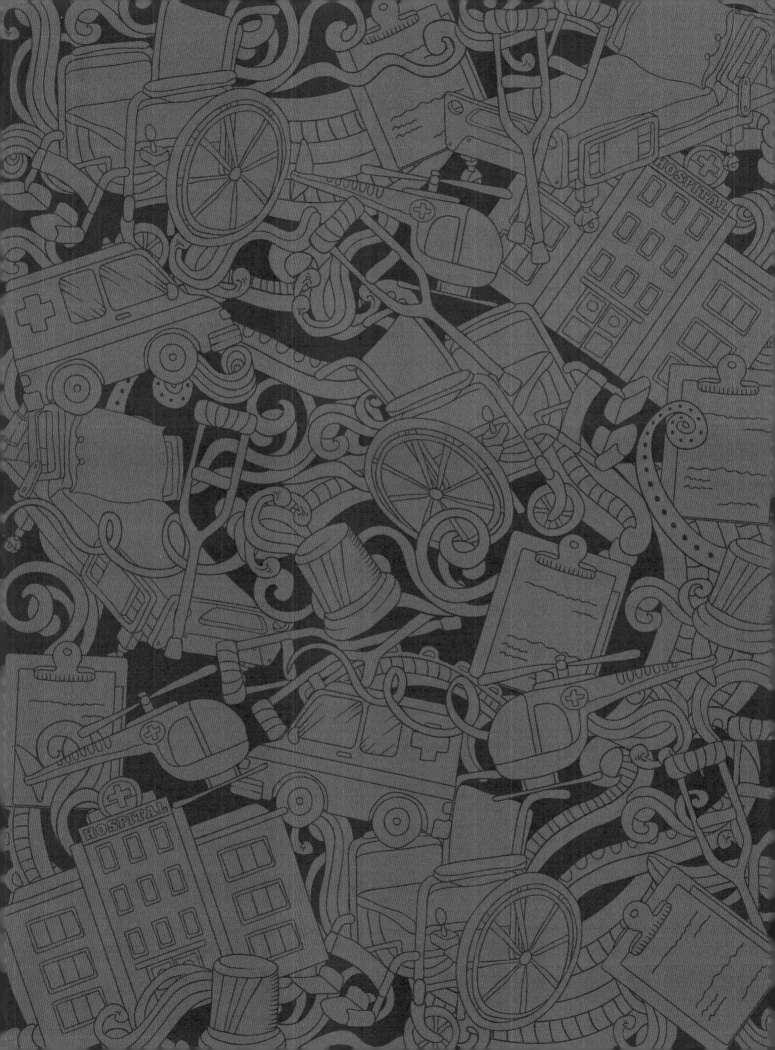

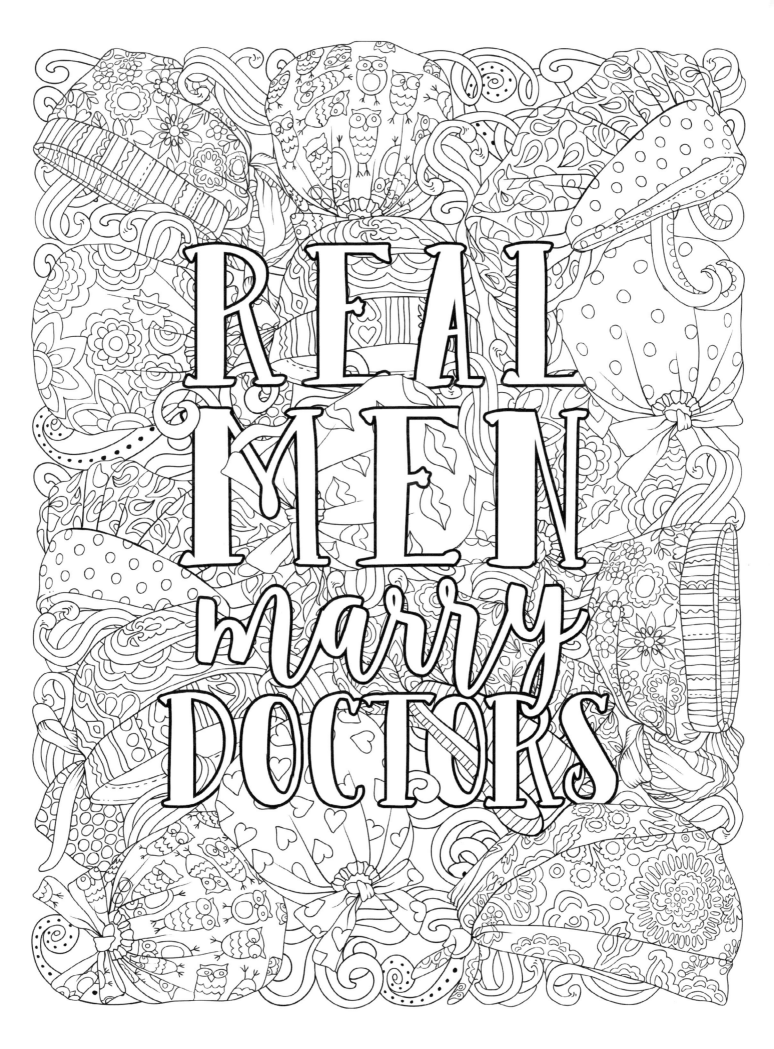

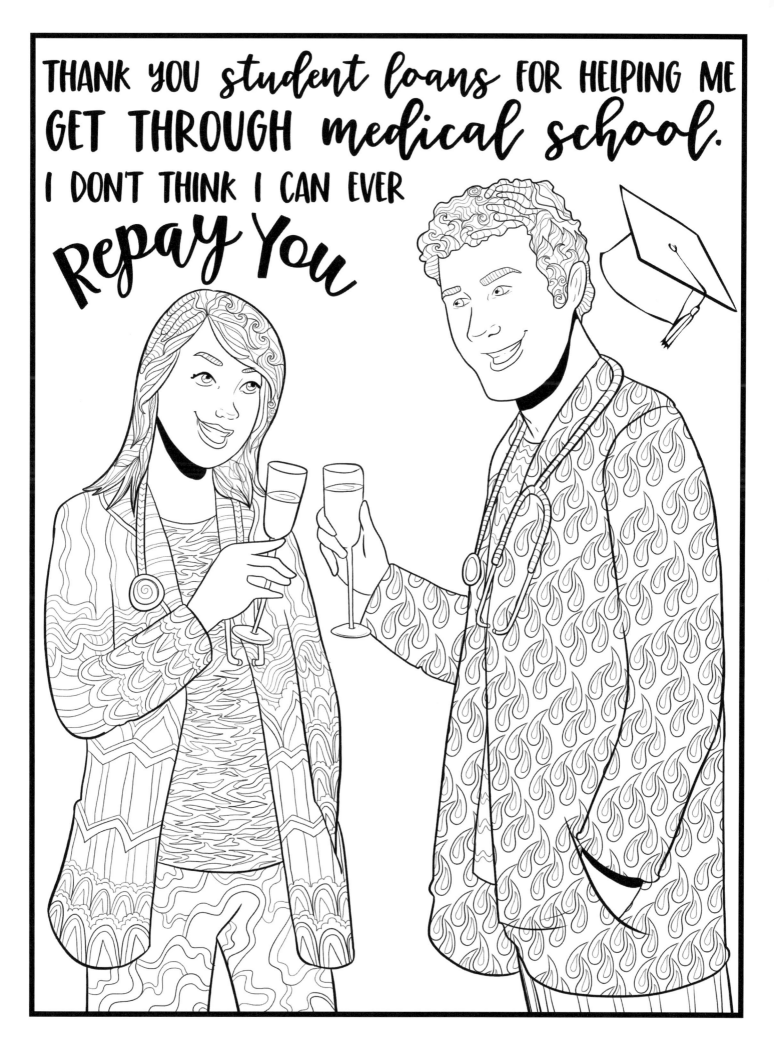

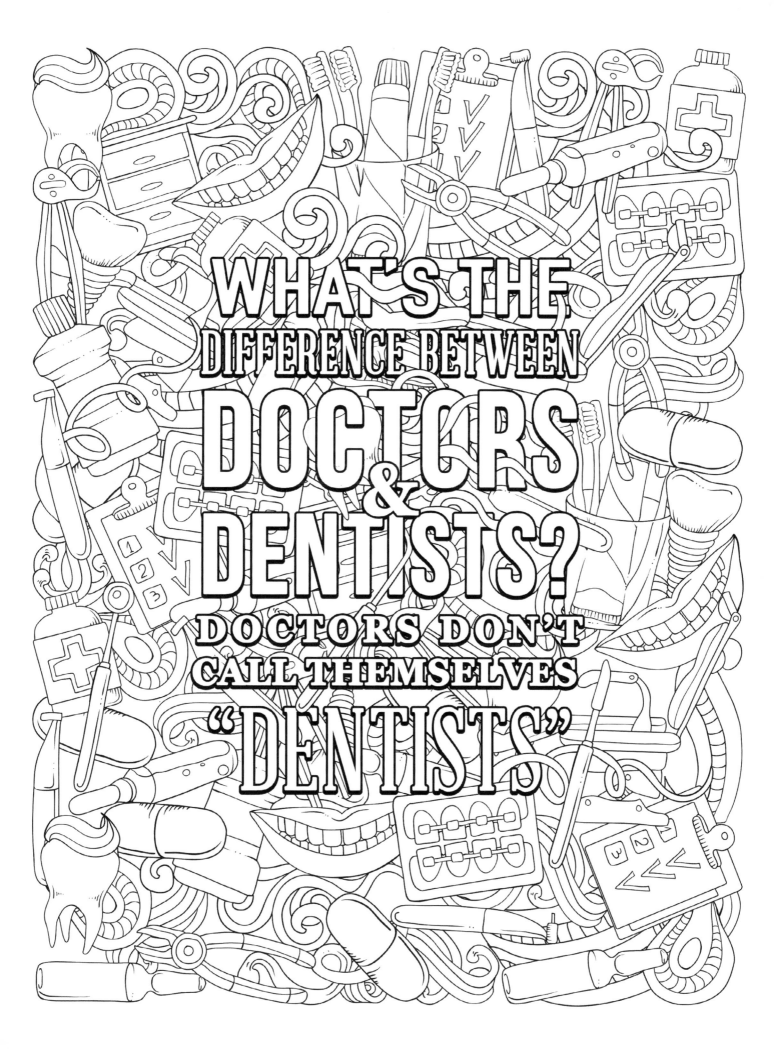

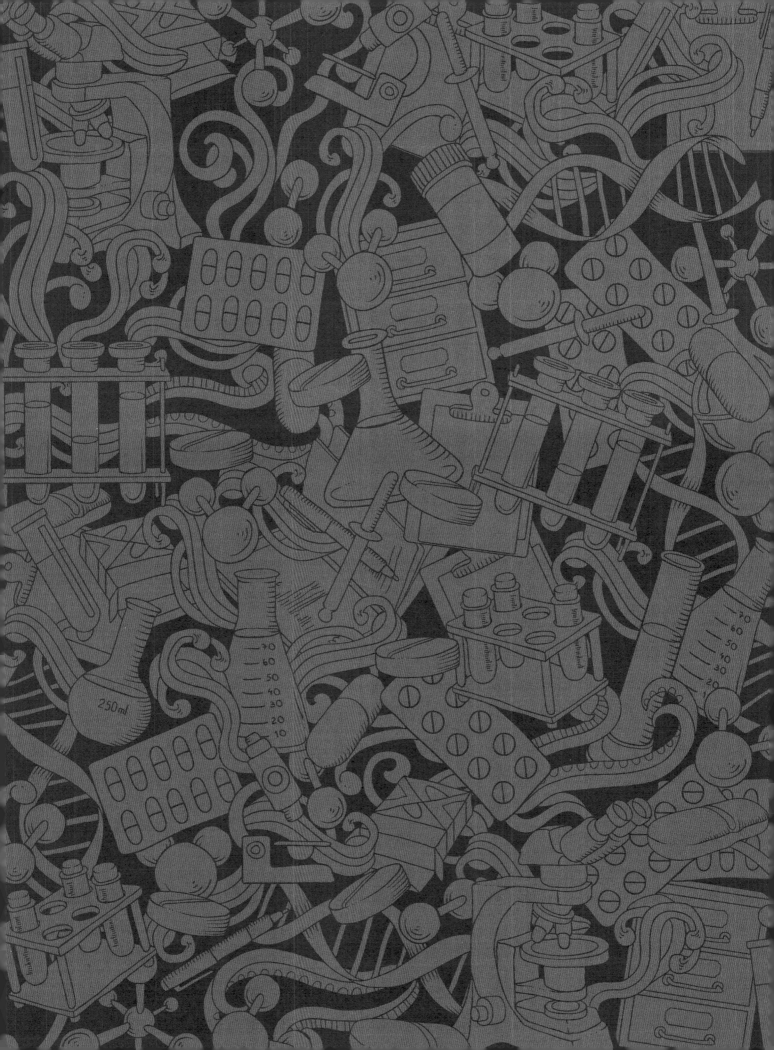

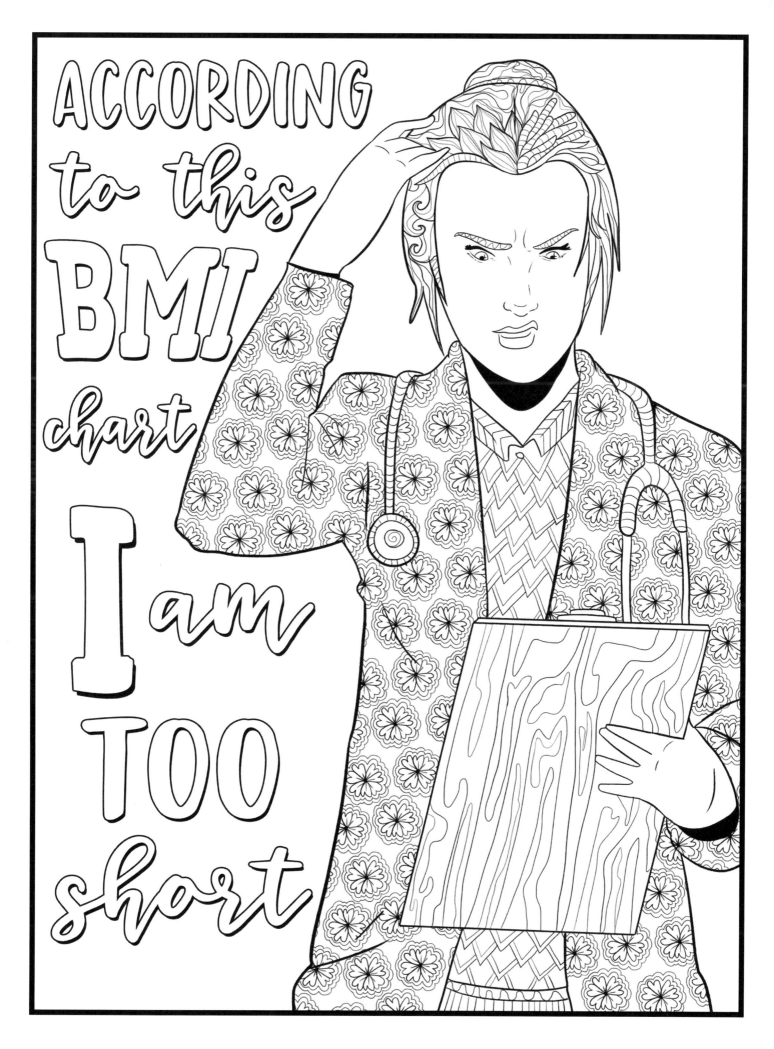

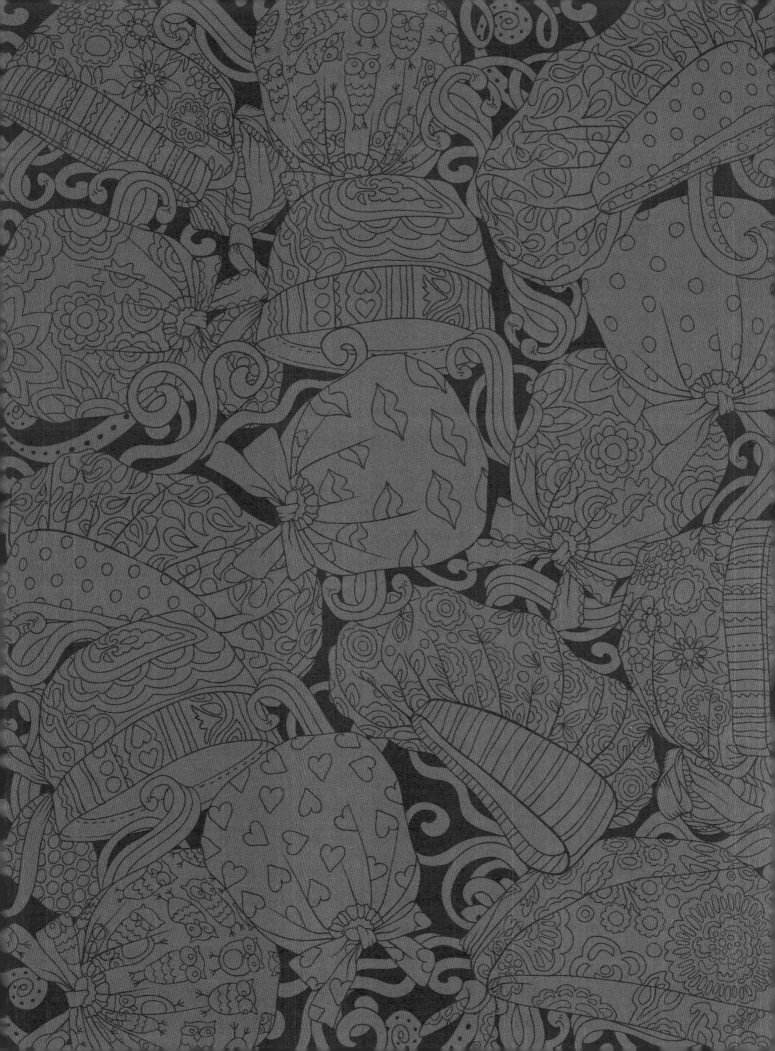

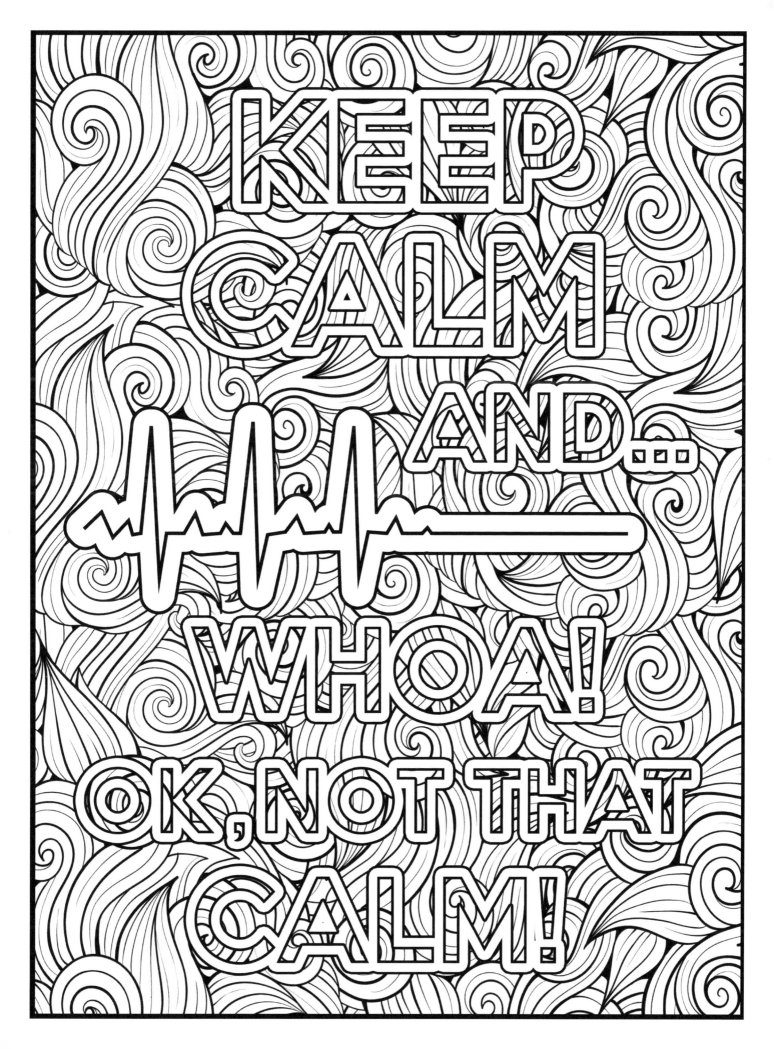

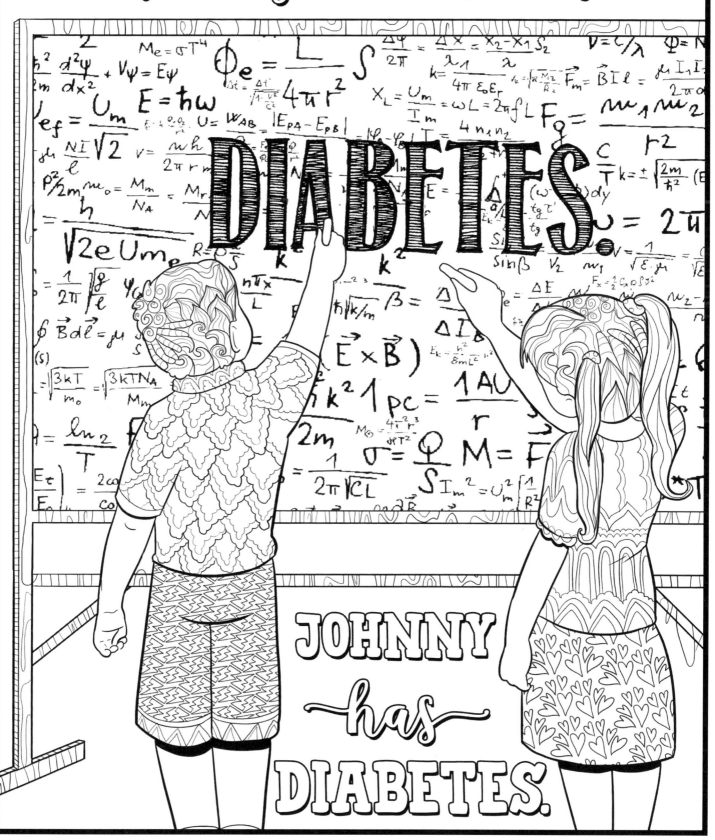

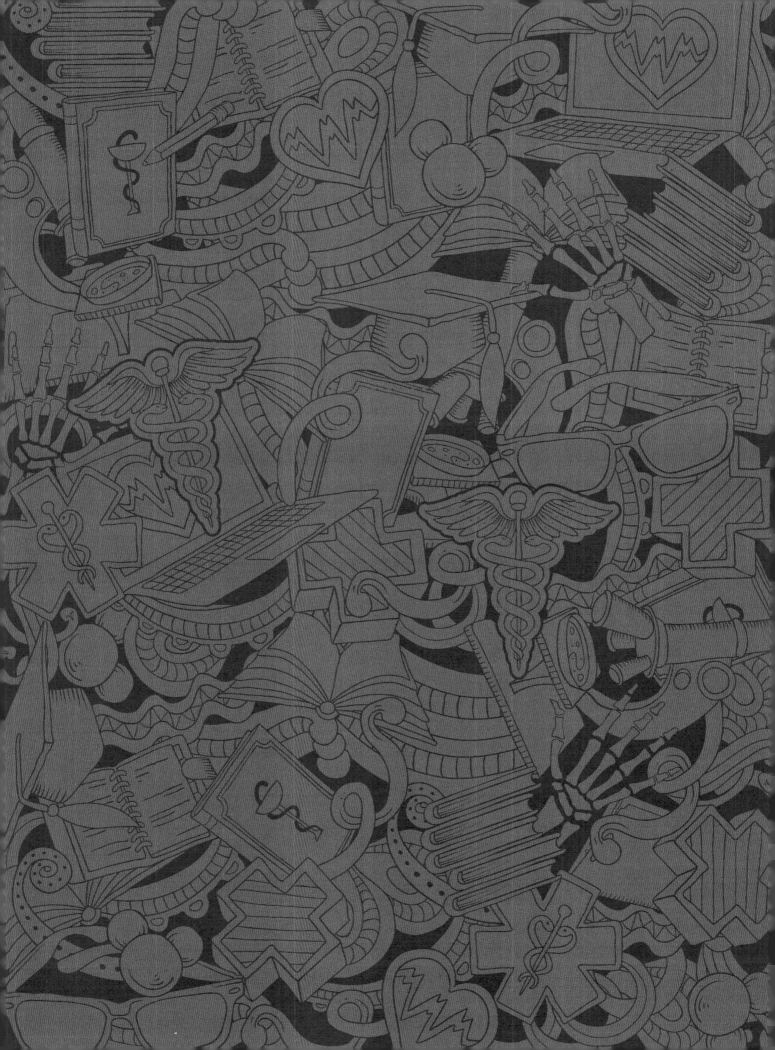

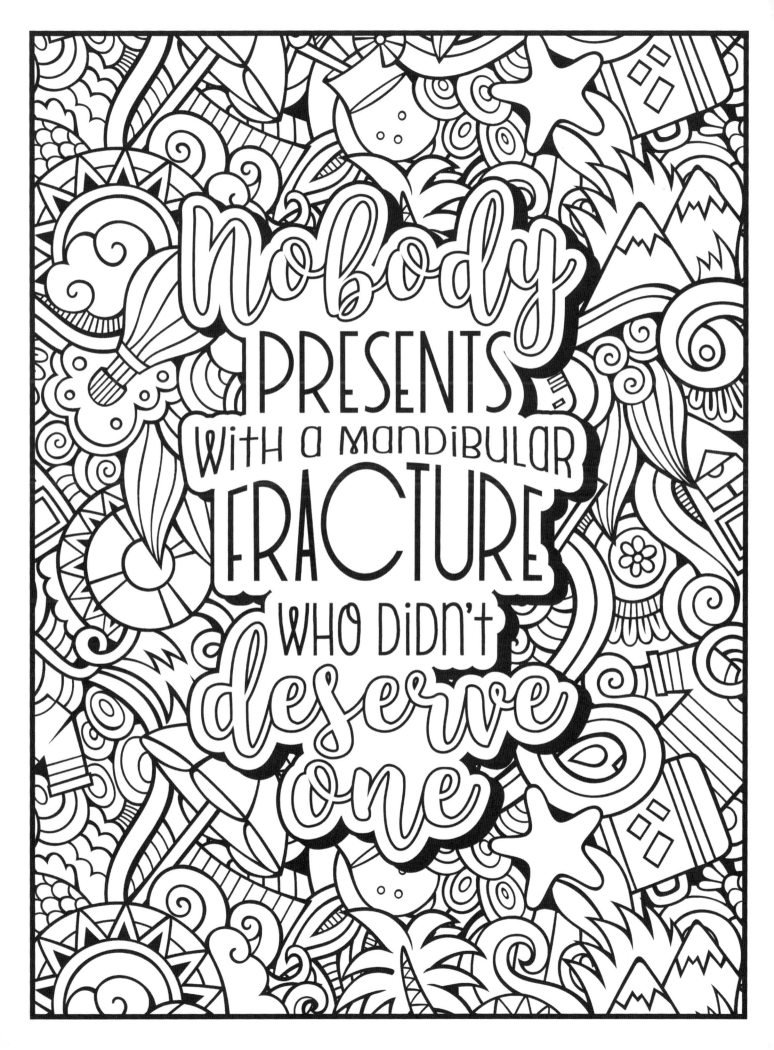

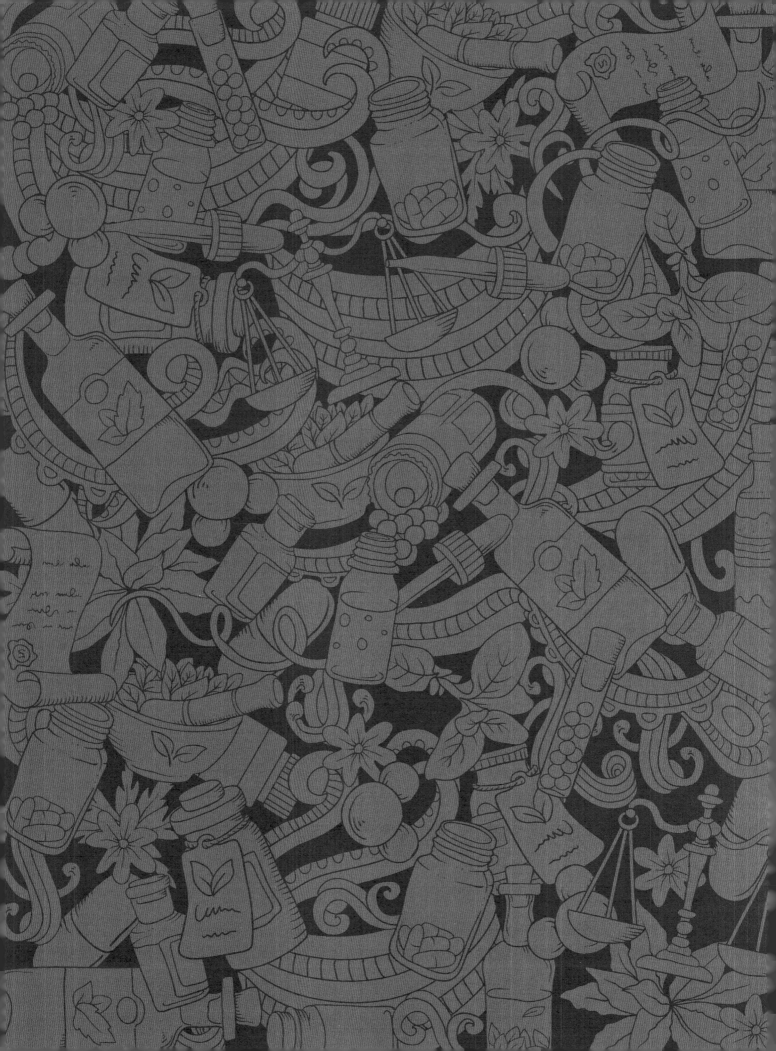

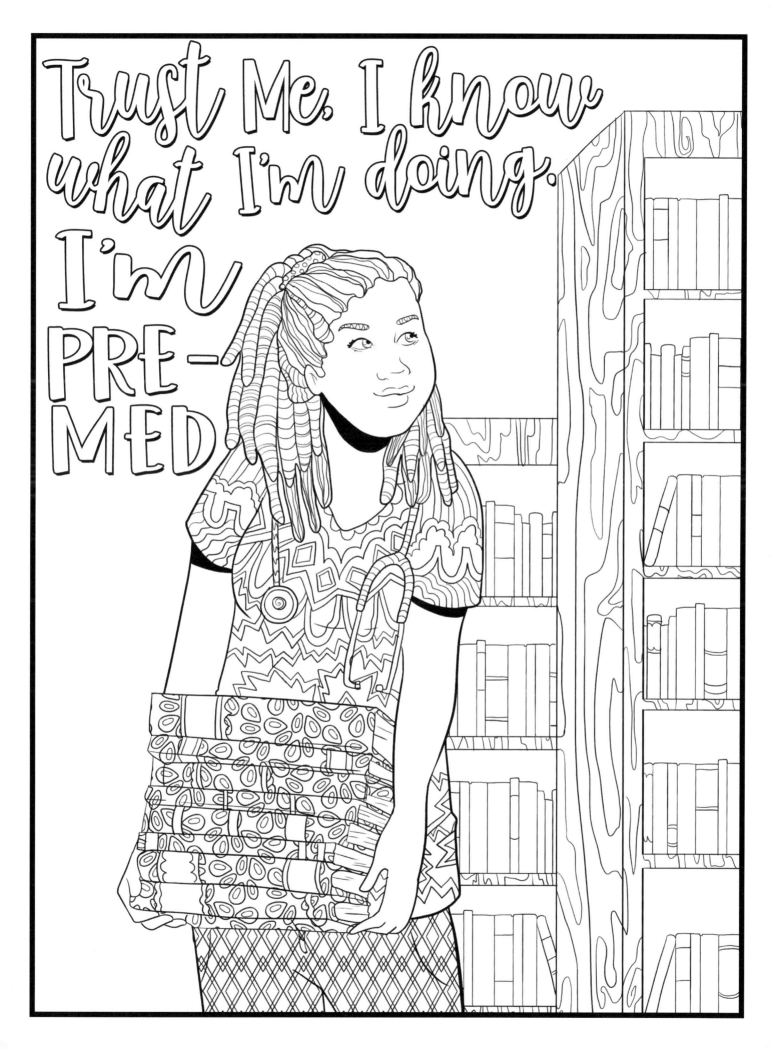

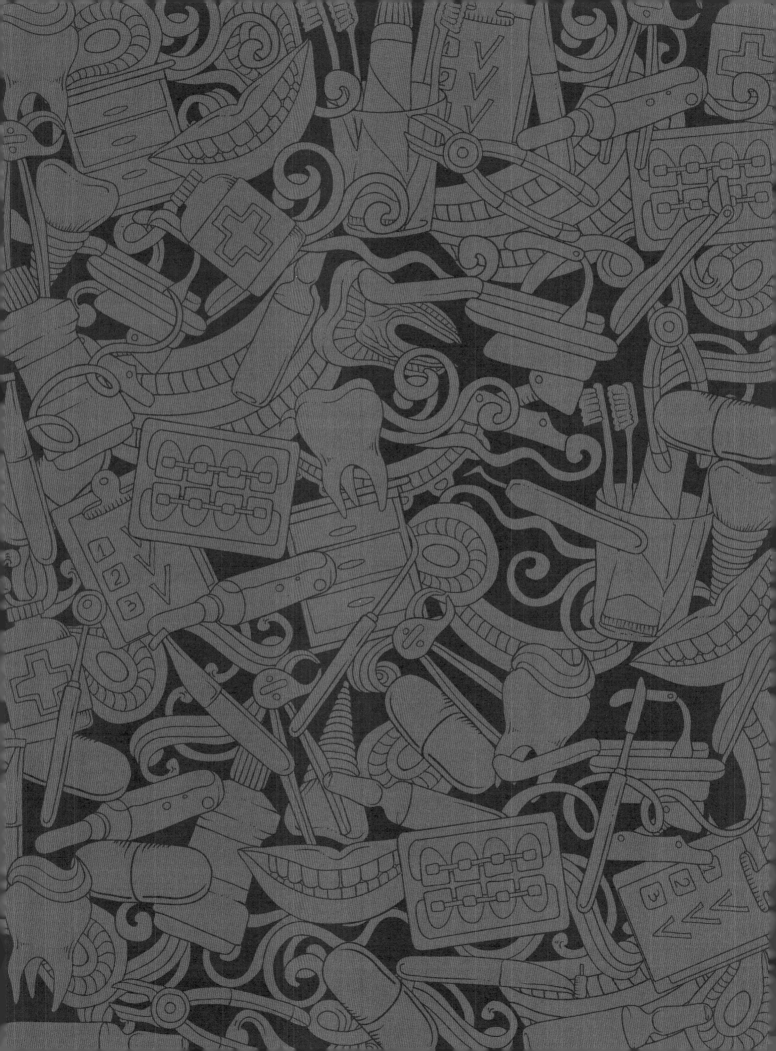

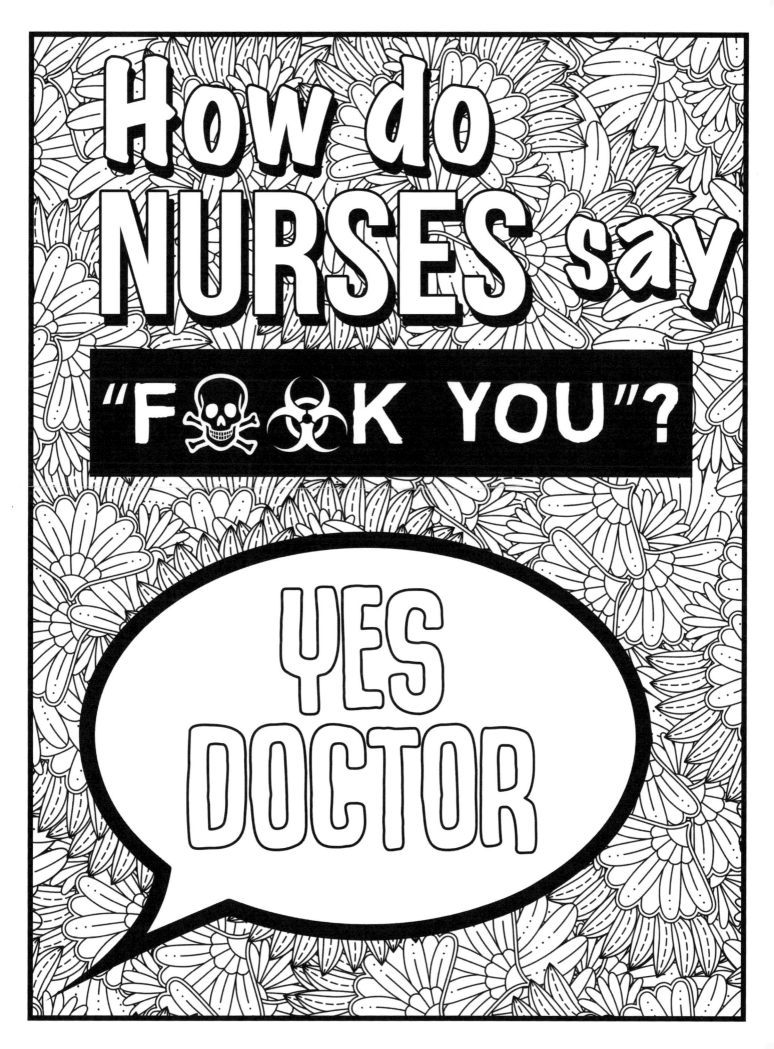

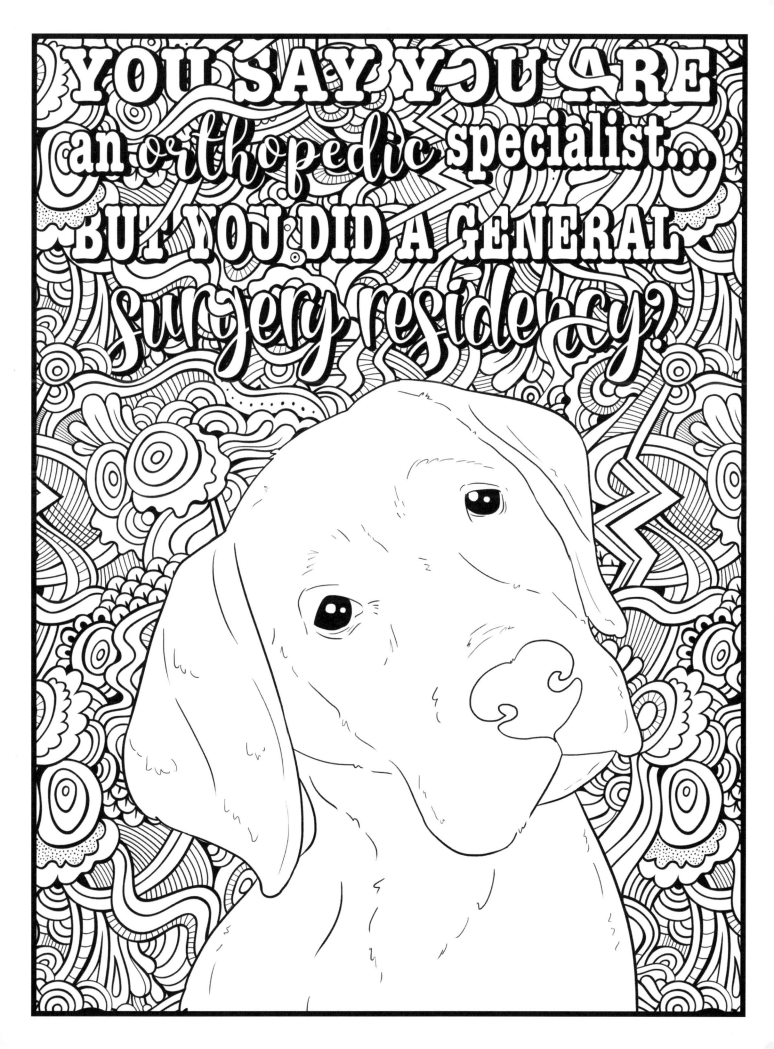

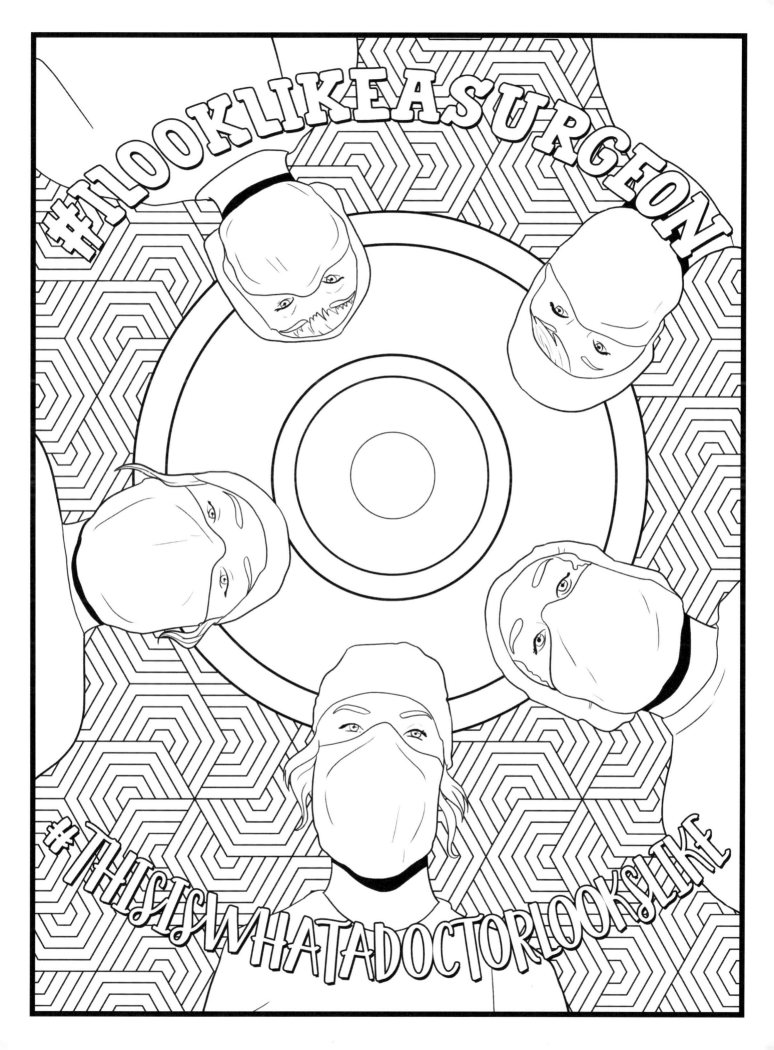

BE SURE TO FOLLOW US
ON SOCIAL MEDIA FOR THE
LATEST NEWS, SNEAK
PEEKS, & GIVEAWAYS

📷 @PapeterieBleu

f Papeterie Bleu

🐦 @PapeterieBleu

ADD YOURSELF TO OUR MONTHLY
NEWSLETTER FOR FREE DIGITAL
DOWNLOADS AND DISCOUNT CODES

www.papeteriebleu.com/newsletter

# CHECK OUT OUR OTHER BOOKS!

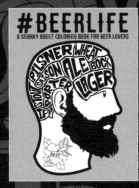

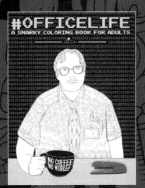

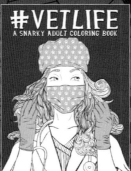

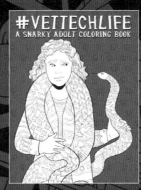

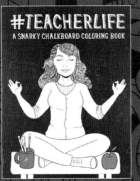

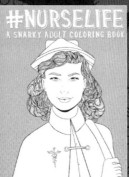

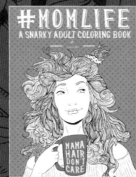

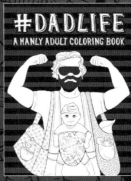

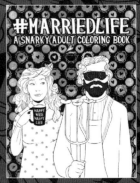

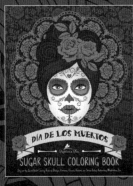

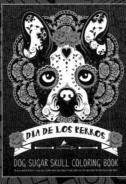

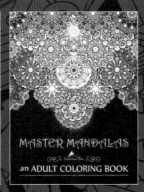

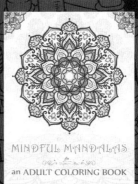

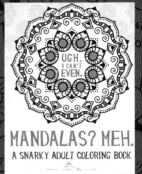

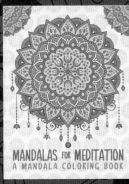

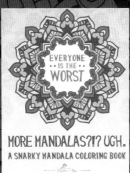

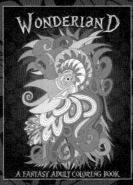

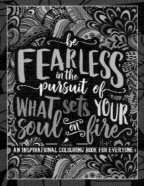

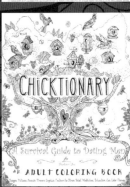

# CHECK OUT OUR OTHER BOOKS!

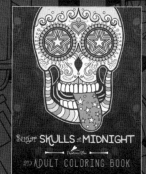

Sugar SKULLS at MIDNIGHT
an ADULT COLORING BOOK

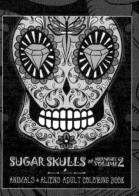

SUGAR SKULLS at MIDNIGHT VOLUME 2
ANIMALS & ALIENS ADULT COLORING BOOK

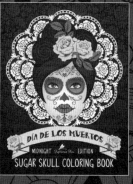

DÍA DE LOS MUERTOS
MIDNIGHT EDITION
SUGAR SKULL COLORING BOOK

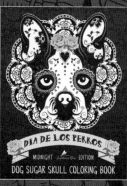

DÍA DE LOS PERROS
MIDNIGHT EDITION
DOG SUGAR SKULL COLORING BOOK

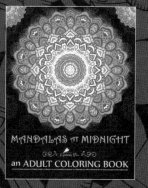

MANDALAS AT MIDNIGHT
an ADULT COLORING BOOK

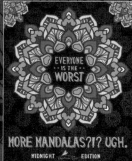

EVERYONE IS THE WORST
MORE MANDALAS?!? UGH.
MIDNIGHT EDITION
A SNARKY MANDALA COLORING BOOK

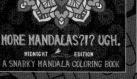

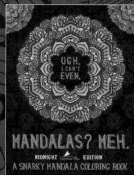

UGH. I CAN'T EVEN.
MANDALAS? MEH.
MIDNIGHT EDITION
A SNARKY MANDALA COLORING BOOK

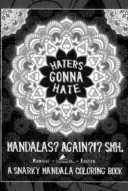

HATERS GONNA HATE
MANDALAS? AGAIN?!? SMH.
MIDNIGHT EDITION
A SNARKY MANDALA COLORING BOOK

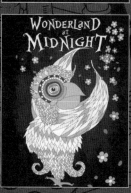

WONDERLAND at MIDNIGHT

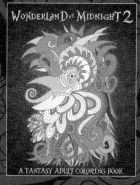

WONDERLAND at MIDNIGHT 2
A FANTASY ADULT COLORING BOOK

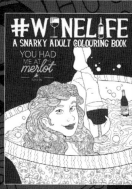

#WINELIFE
A SNARKY ADULT COLOURING BOOK
YOU HAD ME AT merlot

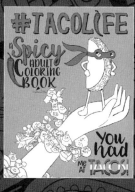

#TACOLIFE
A Spicy Adult Coloring BOOK
YOU HAD ME AT TACOS!

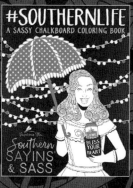

#SOUTHERNLIFE
A SASSY CHALKBOARD COLORING BOOK
Southern SAYINS & SASS
BLESS YOUR HEART

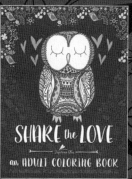

SHARE the LOVE
an ADULT COLORING BOOK

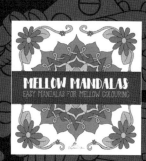

MELLOW MANDALAS
EASY MANDALAS FOR MELLOW COLOURING

# CHECK OUT OUR OTHER BOOKS!

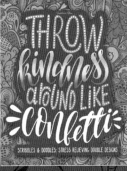

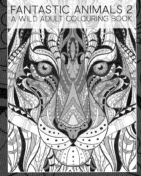

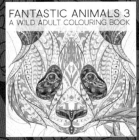

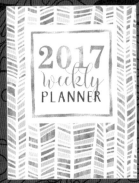

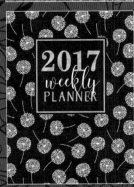

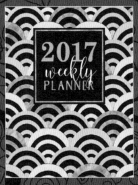

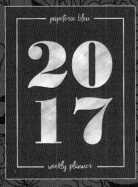

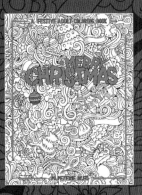

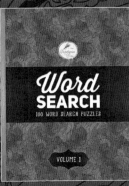

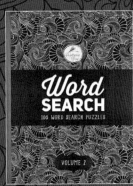

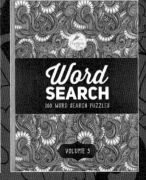

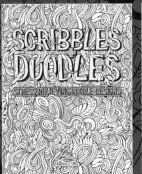

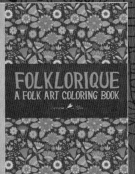

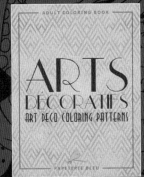

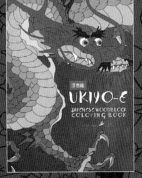

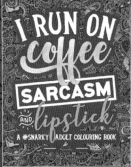

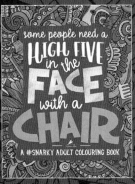

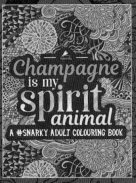